MARY ANN
BYAS-DRAKE

MARY ANN
BYAS-DRAKE

DESTINED *and* DETERMINED
TO BE A NURSE

WILLIS L. DRAKE

Willis L. Drake 9-8-2023

Dedication

THIS BOOK IS DEDICATED TO all of Mary's consanguineous family, particularly her mother, Ruby Smith-Byas, and her father, Mathew Green Byas. The female women in her family that she observed and drew strength from internally (Aunt Mary Tolden, Aunt Biddy (Mildred Thomas), Aunt Francis Anderson, Aunt Alleen Byas, Aunt Margaret Byas, Aunt Allie (Allie Ester Byas-Austin)). As a baseline, Mary's siblings David Byas, Terrence (Terry) Byas, Romona (Mona) Byas-Wooten, and Margaret Ann Byas-Franklin, my "little brothers and sisters" too. This book is also dedicated to you.

Moreover, I hope this book serves as an inspiration to our children and their spouses, Willis Drake Jr., (Marilyn), Monica Renée Drake-Zinn, and Kermit Matthew Drake (Danita), and the next generations of our family (Willis L. Drake III, Adriana Drake-Zinn-Mark, Déjà Renee Drake, and Daren Anthony Lake) and all of my great grandchildren. Above all, Mary's internal strength was that she "had faith in God." She was "Destined and Determined To Be A Nurse."

Table of Contents

Foreword

Romona Byas-Wooten

THERE ARE NOT A TREMENDOUS number of blessings greater than having wonderful sisters. I was blessed to have two, Mary and Margaret. I'd like to tell you about one, Mary Ann. Although her name was Mary Ann, we (her siblings and other family members) lovingly called her Pookie. I'm not sure how this name originated, but she never complained when we insisted on using the designation Pookie.

Since Pookie was some years older than us (her sisters and brothers), we were just children when she married the love of her life, Willis Drake. This union not only began a wonderful journey for them but initiated a marvelous pilgrimage for her siblings—David, Terrance, Romona, and Margaret. They introduced us to experiences (swimming, travel, and meeting new people) that allowed us to blossom. I can vividly remember holidays such as Memorial Day and Independence Day when our Mom and Dad would buy us new outfits to wear. We'd wait excitedly on the porch laughing and playing in anticipation of Willis and Pookie picking us up to go on a picnic, go swimming, or visit other relatives and friends. My younger sister Margaret once wrote to her, "You have made a difference in my life by letting me know that the world is so much larger than just our little, small community where we live. You have shown me by your actions that we should always continue to explore, learn, and grow and that a family that prays together stays together."

My sister was the oldest of five children and always served as our role model. She inspired us by going to nursing school to become a nurse. Seeing her in her nursing cap and uniform was always a pleasure. Not only was she a nurse, but later in life, she went back to school to earn her bachelor's degree. She didn't stop there. She also traveled many miles over the highways in perilous weather conditions to attend Graduate School to earn her master's and become a Doctor's Assistant. By the way, did I mention that she graduated Cum Laude?

Mary/Pookie was special and always made each of her brothers and sisters feel special. However, her efforts did not stop with us; they were extended to our children and our children's children. On several occasions, she planned and completely paid for the young children in the family to go to destinations such as the Ozarks, Chicago, etc. My younger sister Margaret and I went along, and the children and we never forgot the experiences. Ninety percent of the children that went have graduated from college or Nursing School, earned master's, and are striving to be their best.

Interestingly, seventy percent of the children have gone into medical or science fields. Pookie held a very notable place in their lives. You don't have to take my word for it. They have previously stated, "Aunt Pookie, you are one of the strongest people I know, showing not just me but the whole family how to be a success in life on every front, from how you should support and love your family to how you should map out your life from education to God to raising a successful family, you are a true pioneer, and I love you." One of her nieces wrote, "You've always served as a channel for broadening my horizons through the summer trips, testimonies on your nursing career, and inviting Terez and I to the WNBA game with you and your friends. Not every little black girl can say she's been blessed with an aunt like you!"

I guess it's obvious that I love my sister a lot. As a matter of fact, the last time I saw her, my sister Margaret and I realized that Pookie was our "Hero," but Margaret quickly corrected the statement and made it clear that …. No, she was our "She-Ro"!!

MARY (POOKIE), YOU'RE OUR SHE-RO

LOVE, YOUR SISTERS

CHAPTER 1

Destined and Determined (Registered Nurse)!

I VACILLATED BACK AND FORTH AS I considered several scenarios on how to tell my late wife, Mary Ann Byas-Drake's story.

I wasn't sure if I should start Mary's story with her grandparents' life or her parent's life, which greatly influenced Mary, and established the foundation of who Mary Ann Byas-Drake would become. Another option was to start from the first time Mary and I met and what salient information would be pertinent to tell about her life.

I just jumped in the middle of her life story and talked about her intrinsic nature and indispensable qualities. I hope this book will provide some insight into my late wife, Mary's life, portraying predestine, determination, and what is possible under any circumstance.

To begin transferring my beautiful memories of Mary onto the equivalent "parchment paper" to describe her life and essence could be transformative.

Perhaps the steppingstone Mary used to reach her professional achievement of becoming a registered nurse will inspire others. Her grandparents provided her with a living example of hard work and perseverance. Inspiration from her parents to go higher, do better, and set an example for her younger family members coming after her was important. Also, reaching back and helping others in need was an outstanding virtue.

Mary's family members described the nuances of her habits and personality when she was a young girl. Being the only female child in the family living in East St. Louis, Mary was afforded special attention and greater expectations by her family.

From her pre-kindergarten days, Mary was shy and not very vocal. She was reserved in her outward expressions. However, her mother raised her to believe she could accomplish anything she put her mind to achieving.

How many "fire starters" lit the flame of possibility that ignited and illuminated the path of Mary's life that made a difference is unknown. I can name several individuals that aroused and motivated Mary at some point, most importantly, starting with Ruby Smith-Byas, her mother, and Matthew Green Byas, her father. There were other strong women, like her aunts, that encouraged her along her life's path in a direct or subtle way that made a difference in her life.

The lessons she learned from her Aunt, Allie Ester Byas, prepared her to be studious. Being mentored by her Aunt Biddy (Mildred Thomas) taught her to be elegant and professional in her appearance at all times. Being around her maternal and paternal families exposed her to being a caring and loving spirit and individual.

Also, I believe Miss Minnie Edith T. Gore, Homer G. Phillips' Director of Nursing, was spiritually touched as she made an unprecedented exception so Mary could return to nursing school after our first child was born. Also, after our second child was born, Miss. Gore permitted Mary to return and finish nursing school. Mary had witnessed her grandparents endure difficulties through hard work, and now she demonstrated her perseverance in hard work by completing nursing school.

The old cliché "second chance" definitely applied to Mary Ann Byas-Drake's life in the literal sense. As a young teenager and freshman student nurse at Homer G. Phillips nursing school, she could have easily given up on her desire and dreams to become a registered nurse.

However, when adversity stared her (us) in the face, she still believed in her dream and did not flounder. Instead, she became more determined in her desire to be a registered nurse. It begs the question, were the stars in the universe aligned so that the orderly existence of the cosmos would determine Mary Ann Byas' life?

I believe the forecasting of my mother's vision that identified Mary as my wife-to-be three years before I laid eyes on her was a prelude. Thus our marriage, as she and I became one, provided the support Mary required to overcome the interruptions she endured to become a registered nurse.

There were certainly other individuals whom Mary's path crossed that impacted her life, and their actions, regardless of how small, were germane in Mary becoming a registered nurse.

CHAPTER 2

◇

Mother's "Gift" of Visions

◇

IT MAY NOT BE CONCEPTUALLY understandable by everyone; however, I can attest that my mother had a spiritual "gift" of having visions created by the Holy Spirit. When mother had the same vision "three times," it would be manifested exactly as it had appeared to her in the vision.

I have never forgotten that particular Friday evening; it is indelible in my memory. I was coming downstairs from my bedroom on the third floor. When I reached the second floor, my mother stood at the staircase banisher waiting for me. Her facial expression and demeanor were drastically different from her normal effervescent self. She was not smiling, and her body language was tense. Standing there, she was obviously profoundly serious.

The words that came out of mother's mouth were in dramatic fashion. She stated emphatically that "She had this vision three times." She was explicit in her description of the "light brown-skinned girl, a pretty girl." Her facial features were unquestionably clear in the vision, and she would be your wife." Then she said, "Son, watch yourself, you hear."

Standing on the staircase, I was perplexed and amazed at my mother's comments. At sixteen, I did not have a "girlfriend"; most certainly, marriage was as far-fetched as I could imagine. Laughing lightheartedly, I looked up at mother, sort of dumbfounded. Mom, don't worry because I am not thinking about getting married."

She didn't say another word as she turned, walking back to her bedroom. Standing there, I knew mother was earnest about her vision. I also had firsthand knowledge, from past experiences, of my mother's visions being manifested and fulfilled regarding other family members.

I watched mother enter her bedroom, and I continued going downstairs to the first floor. It was Friday evening around 7:15 pm, and I had been in a jovial mood going to hook up with my best friends, James Anderson, and Stanley (Stan) McKissic. We were going to the local teen-town dance in the neighborhood on Taylor Avenue between Washington and Olive Streets, two blocks from my house.

The American Bandstand TV program inspired this "Teen Town Hall" dance craze. I was a junior at Sumner High School, and it was summertime, and the local Teen Town was a place for teenagers to go and have fun on the weekend.

After my mother's comments, temporarily, my enthusiasm waned for just a minute. By the time I left the house, I was refocused on going to the teen town to have fun.

It was unbeknownst to me then that the foundation of my relationship with Mary Ann Byas was rooted in my mother's vision in 1956 when I was just sixteen years old. Little did I know on that particular evening in early September 1959, when I was 19 years old, the impact of my mother's vision would be the mysterious motivation for me walking to Tandy gym. That I then would, in dramatic fashion, meet Mary Ann Byas, a student at Homer G. Phillips Nursing School.

As I began pursuing Mary, getting to know her better, and I established a romantic relationship with her. I didn't have a clue about the connection between my mother's vision three years ago and me meeting

Mary. As our relationship developed, there was a mutual understanding between Mary and I that we care for one another greatly.

Four months later, in December 1959, Mary was on her school's Christmas break. I invited her to my home to have dinner and to introduce her to my mother and family. It was not a formal occasion; we were just going to have leftovers from Christmas dinner. However, I primarily wanted my mother and family to meet Mary.

It was very revealing, as I found out later. When mother first laid eyes on Mary, she immediately recognized her as the "light brown skin girl" that was revealed three years earlier in her vision. It was comical, of sorts, that Mary was being modest, and she didn't accept mother's offer to have something to eat that evening. Maybe she wanted to make a positive first impression by not eating. That was an African-American cultural "thing" that you didn't eat the first time you met someone at their home.

Mary and I sat at the dining room table talking while I ate my food. I teased Mary a little about how good the food tasted. Her constant reply was I'm just not hungry. Mother was in the kitchen for a time, and then she came and sat in the dining room and chatted with Mary briefly.

After I finished eating, Mary and mother said their goodbyes, and I left to take Mary back to the dormitory. Later, I understood that practically before the door closed behind us, mother immediately telephoned her sister Ethel Mae Sanford (Aunt Tee), telling her that Mary was the "light brown skin girl" in her vision three years ago. Mother only confided in her sister, and she never uttered a word to me that Mary was that "light brown skin girl" in her vision.

Mother stated unequivocally, "Ethel, Mary, the young lady that Willis brought to the house this evening for dinner, is the girl I saw in my vision three years ago.""Mary will be Willis' wife in the future." Mother's vision from 1956, when I was sixteen years old, was manifested when she first saw Mary in December 1959 in real life as a guest in her home.

CHAPTER 3

Byas' Family Migration— East St. Louis, Illinois

MARY'S FOREPARENTS, GRANDPARENTS, AND PARENTS were raised in the state of Mississippi. Her father, Matthew Green Byas, was raised in Starkville, and her mother, Ruby D. Smith (Byas), was raised in West Point.

Mary's grandfather Henry Clay Byas (Byars), raised his seven children, four boys and three girls (Henry Drewery Byas; Robertha Byas-Crowder; Allie Ester Byas-Austin; Caldonia Byas-Kemp; Matthew Green Byas; Sterling Napoleon Byas; and Florzell (Flarzell) McKinley Byas) in east-central, Oktibbeha county Mississippi, where he owned over one hundred acres of land in Starkville, Mississippi.

Mary's grandfather also raised farm animals, particularly hogs and cows, and owned a butcher's shop where he sold the meat he processed. Mary's grandfather had the intelligence and forethought to deed the land as "heir property" to retain it within the Byas family. Portions (38 acres) of the land still remain today under Matthew and Flarzell Byas' offspring (Heirs) ownership.

Mary's maternal grandfather Sim Smith (her mother's father) raised his eight children, three boys and five girls (Frank R. Smith, Mary

I. Smith, Lannie C. Smith, Ruby D. Smith, Mildred L. Smith, Sim Smith, Joseph Smith, Frances Smith) in West Point, a city located in Clay County Mississippi.

Without verbalizing it, Mary and I understood our families, the same as many African-American families that lived in Mississippi, Tennessee, and other southern states; they were part of that Great Migration from the south to northern states like Illinois, Michigan, and even Missouri. Their exodus from the south was seeking a better life and opportunities for their children.

With her ever-present effervescent smile, Mary said, "Willis, growing up, I was told that Momma was a very pretty young woman. Her stunning looks attracted my dad big time." Mary was now laughing intently as she said, "West Point and Starkville, Mississippi are twenty-five miles apart. However, that did not dissuade my dad from finding a way to go see momma. He somehow managed to get to West Point to "court" her. I don't know if he traveled by horse or buggy or walked to West Point to see momma, but he got there somehow."

Laughing incessantly, she said, "I am not sure how long my parents dated, but my father was several years older than momma, who was seventeen when they got married. As newlyweds, in 1940, they migrated from Mississippi to East St. Louis, Illinois, hoping for better opportunities to improve their lives. Then I was born a year later after my parents moved to East St. Louis."

I shared with Mary that "my parents moved from Memphis, Tennessee, in 1940, traveling to St. Louis when I was four months old. They had six children, and they aspired to have better opportunities in life for their family and children."

We continued to discuss our historical and geographical similarities regarding our families' common backgrounds. My father was raised mostly in and around Batesville, Mississippi. My mother was raised in Como, Mississippi, a small Panola County town that borders the

Mississippi Delta in the northern part of the state. However, they lived in several areas, including Senatobia and State Line, Mississippi.

Those small towns were within twenty or thirty miles of each other. Therefore, my father had to travel a similar distance to date my mother, the same as Mary's father had to do in dating her mother. I was concealing my laughter. Mary, things have not changed so drastically since then.

My house is probably 10 miles from yours, and you live in a different state than I do. Transportation is more convenient now, but I will find a way to come see you. We both laughed without commenting. However, Mary had a sheepish smile on her face; I'm sure she could relate to the magic or unquestionable feelings when one person's attraction to another person is real.

It did not take much of a stretch to correlate Mary's fundamental innate determination ascribed to that of her foreparents and parents' dogged character, tenacity, and persistence. Early on in her life, the evidence demonstrated that she was destined and determined in whatever she endeavors to do.

CHAPTER 4

Mary's Early Childhood

After Mary's family arrived in East St. Louis, at a point, they lived in "Pollock Town. It was a transitional community where Polish families previously lived, that was now a community where African-Americans were moving into the area. Mary's parents rented an apartment unit in a four-family residential complex at 2209A Kansas Street.

When her family had settled for a year in East St. Louis, Mary Ann Byas was born on Wednesday, October 15, 1941, at St. Mary's Infirmary Hospital, located at 1536 Papin Street in St. Louis, Missouri. There is an African-American cultural saying in my family; "When a baby is born, the Angels visit upon it and forecast what their life will be." The Angels must have stamped on Mary's forehead "destined and determined."

As an infant, Mary's parents nurtured her as she developed into a curious two-year-old toddler. For nine years, she was their only child. Also, at that time, she was the only girl on her mother's side of the family living in East St. Louis. She was appropriately pampered and got special attention from her aunts, and her uncle's favored her as well. Her cousins, Maurice (Sonny) and Alvin Tolden, were boys in the family and were at least four years older than Mary.

Initially, Mary didn't have any playmates at the apartment complex. When Mary was three years old, Ceola Lucas, a girl her age, moved into the apartment complex, and they became best friends. At age four, Marie Morris (Hurst), another girl Mary's age, lived around the corner at 22nd and Broadway. The three girls played together every day and became best friends.

During her preschool years, Mary's parents carried her to Starkville and West Point, Mississippi, to visit their family living there. During her early elementary school years, Mary spent extended time during the summer at her Aunt Allie's home in Starkville. She enjoyed visiting her dad's older sister in the summertime and playing with her cousin Edward, Aunt Allie's son, who was close to her age.

Mary's Aunt Allie was a schoolteacher in the Starkville public school system. When Mary visited her aunt during the summer, she had to read one book a week. Most of the books she read were above her school grade level in East St. Louis. In September, when Mary started school, she was exceptionally prepared for starting her school year in East St. Louis.

When her parents bought a house at 919 11th Street, Mary was six years old. It was on the south side of East St. Louis, a considerable distance from Pollock Town, where they currently lived. Naturally, Mary's parents were ecstatic to buy their own home. However, Mary was less enthused about having to move. Knowing she would be separated from her two best friends, Ceola and Marie left her somewhat devastated at that young age.

Mary's parents settled in their new home and enrolled Mary in Washington Elementary School, where they live. Being naturally shy, Mary was not enthusiastic about attending her new school. She didn't have any friends at school, which was frightening for her.

Juanita Rupert (Russell)

Mary was a second-grader, and her shyness was quite prevailing. On the first day of school, she felt isolated. However, during the morning recess, a classmate with a big smile came and took Mary by the hand, asking if she wanted to play. From that moment, the girl Juanita Rupert (Russell) created an instant friendship with Mary.

Juanita's family lived at 1303 Tudor Avenue, a few blocks from Mary's house. Their families also attended Mount Zion Missionary Baptist Church; Reverend Walter Buford Rouse was the church's pastor, located at 13th and Tudor Avenue. The church was across the street from Juanita's home.

Phyllis McNeese (McReynolds), who was the same age as Juanita and Mary, would visit her grandmother, who lived two houses from Juanita's house. Phyllis and her sister would stay at Juanita's home when Phyllis' grandmother and Juanita's mother went to church choir rehearsal.

Juanita and Phyllis became good friends, and now the three girls, Juanita, Phyllis, and Mary, developed a tight friendship. Phyllis did not live in the same school district and attended a different elementary school than Juanita and Mary.

However, the girls attended the same church, and Phyllis, Juanita, and Mary were Mount Zion Church Youth Choir members. Mary had a unique singing voice and could hit the extra high notes. Phyllis had a beautiful, gifted singing voice, and their youth choir was something special to hear.

Juanita and Mary living only a few blocks from one another, would visit each other's home regularly after school and on the weekends. They were accepted as part of one another's families. The girls were the closest friends, and year after year, it seemed that they had completed elementary and entered junior high school so quickly; but they maintained their very close special friendship.

Mary's uncle, Flarzell, her father's brother, and his wife, Aunt Alleen, lived at 1026 Baker Avenue, within a few blocks of Mary's home. Their daughter Corliss was five years younger than Mary, and they were a close family and visited one another's homes. That was another social outlet for Mary.

Now Mary's young brother, David, was entering kindergarten at Washington Elementary School as Mary was entering high school in 1954. Juanita and Mary entered high school, gripping onto their unwavering friendship. Mary still had a reserved, shy personality, and her social circle did not expand much. Her friendships with Juanita and Phyllis never skipped a beat; it was "solid as a rock."

She was educated in the East St. Louis (public) school District 189 systems. Academically, Mary had punched the right tickets as she went through the secondary school educational system (elementary, junior high, and Lincoln Senior High School).

Mary navigated her high school years, maneuvering through the normal malaise and challenges that high school teenagers encountered. The girls would experience the difficulties that normal teenagers go through growing up. However, whatever it might be, nothing was too monumental for them to "come through it together." Mary loved singing and often participated in Lincoln High School's talent shows.

Mary won singing competitions at school, often performing the song "Fever." That high school experience gave her a degree of recognition from the school's student body, as she gained self-confidence and some popularity from her singing performances.

Mary enjoyed her four years in high school. She did well academically, and her after-school social activities included roller skating, occasional dating, and attending school dances. Now approaching the month of May in her senior year, her high school career would end in a few weeks.

She had enjoyed her high school years as much as any student had. Yet she still remembered the awkward times when she was a freshman and sophomore and did not know her way around the Lincoln Senior High School campus. Mary was not a member of her Lincoln High School "Future Nurses Club." She was a member of the A.V.A. Club (Audio Visual Aid), Junior Classical League, and the Boosters Club.

In her high school classes, her grades were acceptable and exceptional in some cases. She was preparing for college and, subsequently, nursing school. However, her academic grades in mathematics and science were not very substantial.

Following her high school graduation in June 1958, Mary enrolled at Southern Illinois University (SIU) in Carbondale, Illinois, in September 1958. Her focus was to improve her proficiency in mathematics and science and subsequently apply for entry to the Homer G. Phillips School of nursing.

Now, as adults, and after we were married, Mary introduced me to her best childhood friend, Juanita, and her husband, Edward (Ed) Russell. Their friendship always remained intact, although they may not have constantly interacted with one another. When we went to East St. Louis, crossing the Eads Bridge, to the Tudor street exit, periodically, Mary would say, "Willis, Juanita lives there at 1303 Tudor Avenue, and we would stop and say hello to her and Ed.

When we had social gatherings at our home, Juanita and Phyllis and their husbands were always invited, and they attended our parties. In later years when our children were adults, Juanita's daughter Tammy Russell lived and worked in the DMV area (District of Columbia, Maryland, and Virginia).

When Juanita would visit Tammy, she would stay with Mary for a few days and also spend the night at our home during her visit. Observing the two laughing and talking, I would marvel at their true lifelong friendship. I could imagine them as second graders holding hands on the school playground.

It was also astonishing how Juanita's husband, Ed, and I interacted so comfortably with one another and shared common viewpoints on many points of interest. We discussed sports, politics, and the African American historical perspective from our personal experiences. Whenever Juanita, Ed, Mary, and I were together sociably as a couple, we always had fun and enjoyed ourselves.

CHAPTER 5

Homer G. Phillips (HGP) Nursing School

HOMER G. PHILLIPS (HGP) SCHOOL of Nursing was considered one of the country's prestigious nursing schools, particularly among the best African-American nursing schools. There were students from across the United States who sought enrollment at HGP. The admittance of students accepted from within the state of Missouri was naturally higher (75%) than for out-of-state students. Therefore, the out-of-state students, as Mary was, had to be among the top applicants to be admitted to HGP.

After a year of attending SIU, Mary submitted her letter of inquiry to HGP. She had to compete with local Missouri in-state and out-of-state nursing students from across the country that applied to HGP Nursing School.

She completed the testing process and received her admission letter to the rigorous HGP nursing school program. Mary was seventeen (17) years old when she entered the HGP School of Nursing program in August 1959.

There was a limited number of student nursing positions available for each three-year nursing class, and the number of applicants often was four times greater than the student nursing positions available. Mary often said how blessed she felt to be accepted at HGP.

The average class size was approximately thirty nursing students per class. Mary's freshman nursing class had a total of twenty-nine students. Twenty-two were from Missouri, and seven students collectively were from the states of Michigan, Illinois, Arkansas, Tennessee, Mississippi, Texas, and North Carolina.

At 8:00 pm, Sunday night, her parents drove her to the HGP's dormitory before the 11:00 pm weekend school curfew. Her mother reminded Mary with emphasis, "Pookie, if you have any problems, let your Director of Nursing, Miss. Gore know immediately." Mary assured her mother she would contact Miss. Gore if she had any problems.

Mary checked in at the dormitory's registration desk and was informed that her room was on the fourth floor. She hugged her mom and dad goodbye as they left the dorm. Mary was only forty-five minutes from home, where she would spend the weekends away from the school's dormitory campus.

Feeling somewhat melancholy, she quickly unpacked her suitcase and started organizing her items in her room. Hearing voices echoing in the hallway, she went to meet the few students that were in the dorm. Shortly afterward, she returned to her room and ensured that her nurse's uniform was ready for tomorrow morning.

She awakens Monday morning after a restless night's sleep. She took her shower and was dressed by 6:30 am. She and her classmates walked from the dormitory through the tunnel to the hospital cafeteria and had breakfast.

In class on the first day, the instructor provided them with the standard orientation and what was expected of them to complete the program and become a nurse. Her first few weeks of school passed quickly. She adjusted quite well to the HGP's dormitory life, as it was similar to her SIU campus experience.

After her classes in the evening, she and other students had dinner together in the hospital cafeteria. That was when she got better acquainted with her classmates and was able to form some meaningful friendships.

Mary felt comfortable that everything was under control. She knew exactly what her class instructors required of her in the classroom and on the hospital clinical wards. She had also hooked up with a few classmates that were compatible to hang out with sociably.

Meeting Mary Ann Byas
I had been working for four months, and career-wise, everything was looking optimistic for me.

It was late in August, and when I got home from work this particular evening, I laid across my bed to relax. My thoughts wondered for no apparent reason. Then suddenly, subconsciously, going to the Tandy gym at that precise moment was penetrating my thoughts.

It was like a hammer pounding a nail to drive a point home. This impromptu force within me was so strong as if a magnet was pulling me up from my bed, dictating that I go to Tandy gym. I could not rationalize my feelings, so I called Stan (Stanley McKissic), my best friend, to walk with me to Tandy gym.

Stan met me on "the corner," and we walked a completely different way to Tandy gym. It was as if my steps were being guided to take this different and "specific route."

Stan and I were walking and talking, and then we were only two blocks from Tandy gym. Then as if a mirage had occurred, we were at Billy Burkes' restaurant. It was not an optical illusion, as three stunningly; extremely attractive young ladies emerged from the restaurant.

The young lady in the front was looking over her right shoulder, conversing with her two friends behind her. She was oblivious to her immediate surroundings. As I would find out later, this particular evening, she was being exposed by her classmate to a new St. Louis geographical area, commonly known as the "Ville"; and to "Billy Burkes," the best hamburger place in the city.

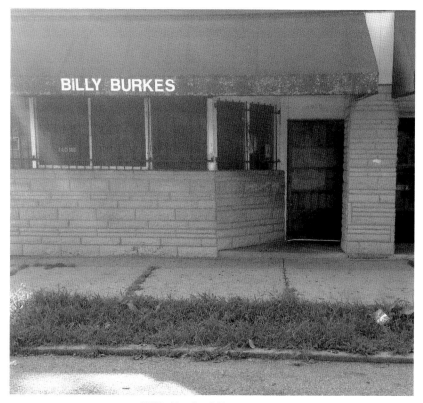

Billy Burkes' Restaurant

Walking out of Billy Burkes', this young lady practically bumped into me. I stopped abruptly, inches from physically colliding with her "stacked physique." She was now standing on the sidewalk. I composed myself, but I was instantly mesmerized as we were face-to-face in close proximity to each other.

I was captivated by her. There was a shyness about her "saying I am sorry, please excuse me." She asked, are you okay? Stopping so abruptly can be jarring sometimes. I assured her that I was fine. She had an unbelievably soft voice, and the tone of her words sounded contrite and sincere. Her voice immediately caught my attention, which was another attraction that propelled me to want to know her.

There are many words that could apply in explaining our meeting. Was it happenstance, serendipity, fate, destiny, or predestined? Based on my mother's vision, I choose to believe that it was predestined that we were to meet on this day.

I cast my eyes on her, and following my male instincts, I quickly observed that she was wearing black Bermuda shorts that fit her just right! Immediately her physical attributes were very obvious to me. I observed that she was about five feet two inches tall and weighed about 115 pounds. She was built very nicely, and she had big pretty legs. Her hair was cut medium short, and she had a beautiful, inviting smile. In the vernacular, and in my opinion, this young sister was "positively fine," period.

Inconspicuously, the three eye-catching attractive young ladies, and Stan and I, in the natural sense, were checking each other out. I then recognized Connie (Constance Fitzpatrick), who I knew from the Tandy dances when we were in high school. She graduated from Beaumont High and I from Sumner High.

I had not seen her in over a year. We exchanged the normal "how have you been? It is good to see you dialogue." I asked in the normal flow of our conversation, "what are you doing in this area, and who are your friends?" She laughed and said, "Willis, I brought my friends to Billy Burkes' to taste the best hamburgers in the world." Stan and I have eaten plenty of Billy Burkes' burgers and confirmed they were the best in the city.

With my eyes on this particularly fine sister, "I asked Connie to introduce her friends." She quickly made that sisterhood non-verbal eye contact with her companions to ascertain their approval or not.

Then responding quickly, she said, "sure, we are classmates attending Homer G. Philips' Nursing School. Willis, this is Grace Adams and Mary Byas; he is Willis Drake, but I don't remember your friend's name. "Oh, this is Stanley McKissic, my best friend. Grace and Mary, we are glad to meet you."

This young lady that I was mesmerized by was a freshman student in her third week as a member of the 1962 Homer G. Phillips nursing school class. It was a few months before her eighteenth birthday. Coupled with getting her nurse's training, she was also being exposed to a vast new social and cultural environment of eighteen to twenty-one-year-old young women from various nationwide backgrounds.

The nursing students lived in a five-story dormitory. The HGP's medical facility was staffed by African-American doctors, nurses, technicians, and administrators. When the hospital was established, Homer G. Phillips was one of only two medical institutions where African-American doctors could receive medical training. The hospital also provided accommodations for treating six hundred (600) in-house hospitalized patients.

It is difficult to imagine, unbeknownst to me, that possibly some unexplainable force, on this particular day, required me, without any preconceived intentions, to walk to Tandy gym.

Concurrently, little did Mary Ann Byas know that her cultural exposure to one of the local African-American restaurant/hamburger establishments would be paramount to our meeting at this precise time. Sometimes as individuals, we can never ascertain where or how our paths will cross with one another. We could only assume or ask whether it was predestined or a serendipitous meeting.

The five of us were suspended in time, standing in front of Billy Burkes' talking gaily with one another. I asked Mary and Grace if they enjoyed eating Billy Burkes' burgers.

They both responded, "Yes, those burgers were good." Mary said they put a lot of onions on their burgers, just how I like mine." Mary, I like lots of onions on my burgers too. We have something in common already." We both laughed as it was obvious we were checking one another out.

I was not sure what would come next. Then Connie said, "Willis, we have to get back to the dorm. We still have to study tonight. It is good seeing you, and I hope to see you again soon."

I definitely wanted to talk to Mary and did not want this opportunity to pass me by. I asked, "can we walk you'll back to the dorm just to make sure you get there safely?" It was a humorous moment, and we all laughed. With their unified concurrence, "Sure, that will be fine."

Cool, and looking at Mary, I declared, "I will be your personal protector walking you back to your dorm." My humor generated laughter from the young ladies, and Connie said, "excuse me. Mary go on, girl; you must have impressed. Having Willis as your "personal protector is an honor."

I said, "Stan and I were initially on our way to Tandy gym." Then Connie suggested, "We walk by Tandy on the way back to the dorm. It's only one more block to walk, and we can use the exercise after eating those burgers."

As Mary and I walked towards Tandy, there was unexplained chemistry among us. We were having a lighthearted conversation, walking, talking, laughing, and enjoying the evening as newly acquainted young people.

I learned that Mary and I were compatible in our interests and temperament. We were also interacting as if we had known each other for a long time. Our conversation flowed spontaneously as if the words were being orchestrated between us.

Weather-wise, it was a pleasant evening to walk, and we passed Sumner High School. I told Mary that was my alma mater that I graduated from last year. As we turned the corner at Pendleton and Kennerly Avenues, we were one block from the Tandy Gym.

The Retaining Wall

The Sumner High School football practice field covered three-fourths of the block, and the Tandy Center was the only building on the block.

It was now just before dusk. With the city streetlights shining on her, I could see Mary's face and that pretty smile more clearly. We were approaching the retaining wall that kept the "ground soil" from washing off the practice field when it rained. The retaining wall was a stone and concrete structure about one foot wide and three feet high at the apex.

Mary and I had met just fifteen minutes ago, and obviously, she was acting playful and a little silly too. She started walking on the small retaining wall, and it just blew my mind. This being the first time we met, it was amazing how naturally comfortable she was with me. She was a confident young woman, and that got my attention.

She was walking with her arms extended out from her body like she was balancing herself on a high wire tightrope in a carnival act. She was being dramatic, laughing, and obviously enjoying herself.

Here we were, two mature young adults acting like young kids. Stan, Grace, and Connie turned around to see Mary walking on the retaining wall and started laughing. However, with astonishment in her voice and a surprised look on her face, Connie said, "Mary, come on, girl. You are acting like a little kid. Don't embarrass me like that in front of Willis and Stanley."

We were laughing like young adolescents. Then, with a little attitude in her voice, Mary said, "Connie, excuse me, I am not acting like a kid! I am sorry if it embarrasses you that I am enjoying walking and talking to Willis." I was smiling as I chimed in and said, "Connie, do not worry. Mary and I are doing fine. You, Grace, and Stan just keep walking."

Connie said, "Okay, I guess you told me; I will shut my mouth." The laughter roared louder as we continued walking toward the dorm at Homer G. Phillips.

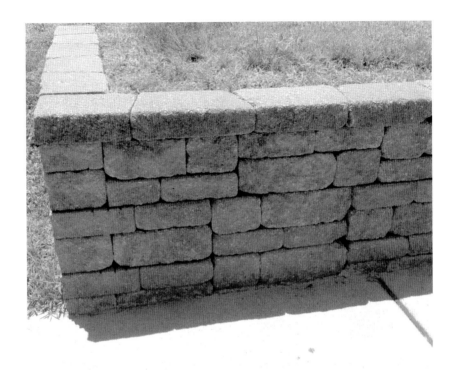

The Retaining Wall

However, as Mary was walking on that retaining wall, she was two feet higher than I was. In view of the illuminated streetlights, I was able to capture a full view of Mary's statuesque figure. I could see that, yes, she was fine! I was observing her physical attributes, her build, and her big, pretty legs most of all. Which were accentuated very well by her appropriately fitted Black Bermuda shorts. I was getting a full view of this fine, healthy young sister. I was becoming impressed by her appearance, personality, and engaging conversation. Smiling to myself, I thought, *Girl, you bad with your fine self.*

As I looked up at Mary on the retaining wall, my male player's instincts kicked in automatically. I asked to hold her hand so she wouldn't fall, and without hesitation, Mary reached out and gave me her left hand. As we walked toward the Tandy Gym, Mary was still walking on the retaining wall, and I was holding her hand.

I had been holding her hand for about two or three minutes when we got to the end of the retaining wall. Mary then gave me her right hand, and I helped her down to the sidewalk. I honestly believe that was the exact moment Mary and I spiritually and romantically clicked. When I asked Mary, "Let me hold your hand," she reached out her hand to me, and I held it.

I believe that simple connection, holding hands, instinctively cemented our future together. I think symbolically and factually, that was the fulfillment of my mother's vision that the Holy Spirit had shown her three times three years earlier when I was 16 years old.

We were now at the dormitory, and Mary and I lingered for a few minutes before we said goodbye. Then Stan and I headed back home. Ironically, Stan did not have any further contact with Grace, nor did we stop by Tandy gym that evening. Apparently, the purpose and inspiration for me going to Tandy gym was to meet "Mary Byas, " which was accomplished.

Two days later, I made "the call," and our first phone conversation was cool. I wanted to know if the chemistry from a few nights ago was still apparent. Initially, there was some vagueness of not knowing exactly what to talk about, but the conversation started to flow well later. At one point, Mary said, "Willis, some of my classmates went to Sumner High School, and they know you."

My ear was pressed tightly against the phone's earpiece. In that soft voice, Mary let me know she was checking me out with some classmates. Therefore, I assumed she must have some interest in me. I had anticipated having this first phone conversation, and I sensed that Mary was also anticipating talking to me.

With curiosity, I asked, "what did your classmates say about me?" With a chuckle, she said Willis, what do you think they said. Then laughing, she responded in a matter-of-fact way. They said, "You are a nice and pretty cool guy." I let her words marinate for a moment in silence. I was immersed in the thought of her classmates' high endorsement of me as a person.

Mary broke the silence by saying, "Willis, when we met, my first impression was that you are a nice person." I assured her that you are a good judge of character and I am a nice guy. Mary, my impression is that you are a lovely person also.

Our first conversation was not long; however, the chemistry from our first meeting still existed. There was no gamesmanship being played by either of us. We talked about our social interests, the type of entertainment and music we enjoy listening to, and Mary enjoyed roller skating.

As we ended our conversation, I asked Mary if she wanted me to call her again. Responding without hesitation, "Yes, Willis, I enjoy talking to you. You can call me tomorrow evening at this time. I will be finished with my dinner then." Okay, I will call you tomorrow, and we said goodnight.

Our Telephone Conversations Continue

I called Mary the following night, and we talked during the next week and a half every evening. We spoke freely about virtually everything, and our telephone conversations were our modus operandi.

The depth of our conversations did not change. In less than a few weeks, the connection between Mary and I had evolved tremendously. I was a good listener when she had a rough day, and she could vent her emotions to me. On those difficult days, after talking, she would be uplifted and encouraged. We connected extremely well emotionally, considering we had only known each other for a brief time.

I had flings with girls in high school, but I never had a serious romantic relationship in high school with any one particular girl. Now I had this emerging and developing relationship with Mary that I was interested in cultivating to the fullest. For over a week, we had engaged in nightly telephone conversations, and I wanted to see Mary again.

I asked Mary if I could come to see her next week after I finished my gym workout. She said, "Yes, Willis, can you come Wednesday at 8:00 o'clock? I will be finished eating dinner, and my studying will be out of the way by then; we can visit for a while." I was gleeful as I let her know, yes, Mary, 8:00 o'clock Wednesday will be cool for me.

That was spot-on as we said goodnight. I retreated to my bedroom lounge area to listen to my R & B music. I was totally relaxed and meditating with the music in the background, thinking of Mary. Shortly after that, I went to bed and fell asleep.

Our Relationship Intensifies

Wednesday was here, and after work, I went home, and within an hour, I went to the gym as usual. I had an exhausting workout that evening. It was ten minutes to eight as I was heading to the HGP dorm. Although I was physically spent, I was excited to see Mary when I left the gym.

This would be the first time I would cast my eyes on her since that unexplainable meeting we had over a week ago. The image of how fine Mary looked in her black Bermuda shorts was permanently etched in my mind.

The dormitory was at 2516 Goode Avenue (Annie Malone Dr.), and it takes less than five minutes to walk there from Tandy Center. I was fatigued when I reached the dormitory, but I gathered my composure and entered the building. Mary had explained the visitors' protocol process for visiting a student nurse to me.

She said Mrs. Gilkey (Bertha) is really nice, and she probably would be on duty at the front desk." However, Ms. Clark might be on duty, and the students have dubbed her "sergeant-at-arms." Mary laughed; Willis, I wouldn't know because you are my first visitor. When you sign into the visitor's registration book, I will get a call (buzz) from the front desk, and I will come down to the lobby.

Entering the dormitory lobby, I saw the receptionist whose name tag was Mrs. Gilkey. Immediately I understood why Mary would like her. She was smiling and asked, "May I help you, young man?" Good evening; I came to visit Mary Byas. Can you please let her know Willis Drake is here to see her?"

The visitor's protocol was professional and secure, yet it had a sense of parental concern with Mrs. Gilkey's presence. She asked me to "Sign my name in the visit's registration guestbook, and please wait in the visitor's lounge for Miss. Byas." I was impressed by this totally first-class nursing institution, Homer G. Phillips.

I waited for Mary, a future nurse, to be produced from this African-American hospital nursing school, HGP. At the time, I was unaware of the historical significance of Homer G. Phillips hospital and its value to the African-American community in the "Vile" in St. Louis. I am not sure why, but I felt proud waiting for Mary to appear in the visitor's lounge.

I was hoping Mary would appear quickly as I was feeling physically exhausted, and I did not want to doze off waiting for her. It had been ten minutes, and I recall the exact moment she walked into the visitor's lounge. Seeing her, I thought my mind was playing a trick on me. She wore this alternating brown and white full-pleated checkered "three-inch square pattern" skirt with an oversized baggy top. She looked kind of plump.

My first mental reaction was, "wow," she doesn't look the same as that fine young lady I remember meeting just days ago. I had this physical image of Mary wearing those black Bermuda shorts and that beautiful smile on her face.

Apparently, my facial expression caught Mary off guard. As she walked closer to me, she had a puzzled look on her face. Then she leaned down, her face was close to mine, and our noses were practically touching. Mary's spontaneous reaction, at that moment, "thawed my frozen irrational brain."

Then in her sweet soft voice but in a questioning tone, she said, "What's wrong, Willis? You are not glad to see me?" She then smiled. Immediately, I could see her personality surface and that beautiful smile adorn her face. Suddenly, I was able to visually recapture the "fine sister" that I was smitten by just days ago.

The emotional connection and physical attraction we experienced when we first met now totally emerged. Our eyes glazed on one another for the second time. It was obvious that the "romantic juices" was still present, and I engulfed the moment."

Mary and I had the visitor's lounge to ourselves, and we sat in the corner of the lounge. We talked, laughed, and had fun for forty-five minutes. My earlier fatigue when I entered the dorm seemed to dissipate but not totally disappear. I enjoyed my visit with Mary and could tell the feeling was mutual. Being with her triggered excitement, and we had a super visit together.

I never thought about her baggy clothes again. I was mesmerized by her sweet soft voice, beautiful smile, and us just clicking as we talked. Reluctantly, I told Mary I needed to go and asked: "if she would call me a taxicab."

She was serious but teasingly said, "Willis, I have finished studying, and my curfew is not until 10:15, and I have over an hour before curfew if you want to stay longer." I admitted, "if I stayed longer, I might fall asleep on you." We laughed, and Mary left and called me a taxicab. Within a minute, she returned and said the taxicab would arrive shortly.

We were now standing alone in the lobby facing each other, and I was unsure how we would say goodnight. Circulating in my mind, I thought, "was it too soon to kiss Mary goodnight? Would it be appropriate for me to give her a polite hug goodnight?" These thoughts penetrated my mind. However, the issue was resolved without question.

Standing alone in the visitor's lounge, we looked into one another's eyes; it just happened. It was spontaneous, as we kissed lightly, but it was not a lingering kiss. It was just perfect! We said goodnight as the taxicab pulled up in front of the dorm. Mrs. Gilkey and I also said goodnight as I departed the dormitory.

I waved bye to Mary as I literally crashed into the backseat of the taxicab. I had forgotten all about feeling exhausted and having sore muscles. I had a wonderful time with Mary, laughing and talking like we had known one another for a long time.

I gave the cab driver my address, and I knew I would be home in twenty minutes. Then I thought about "the goodnight kiss." I was now nestled in the backseat of the taxicab anticipating a relaxing ride home.

When the taxicab pulled up in front of my house, I paid the driver and exited the cab. Entering the house, suddenly I was feeling tired again. It was nine-twenty, still early, but the TV was off, and no one was downstairs. I went straight upstairs to my bedroom.

My mind wandered back to my visit with Mary. Thinking of her at this point, just for a minute, my physical exhaustion had escaped me. Now in my bedroom, I reverted to my usual routine. However, instead of my jazz music, I turned on the radio to listen to my favorite Deejay, Dave Dixon (radio station KATZ), playing some "bad sounds" R&B music as I lay across my bed.

I now was visualizing Mary's beautiful smile, soft voice, and the laughter and enjoyment we had shared this evening. The sincerity of her asking me to stay longer confirmed in my mind that she, too, had enjoyed seeing me. Then our goodnight kiss was a seal of approval that Mary and I wanted to see one another again, and most likely, we would pursue developing a meaningful relationship.

Now lying in bed and listening to the music, I reminisced for a brief time and was completely knocked out. I slept soundly until I woke energized the next morning, with the radio still on. I got up refreshed, with a feeling of gusto. I bathed, got dressed, and I had pep in my step, more so this morning, getting ready for work and waiting for my ride.

I rode to work with my friend Cleart Jones, who charged me bus fare, and the money helped pay for gas for his car. As friends, we talked about the girl in our lives. When I got in the car, I was grinning profusely; however, I wanted to act cool.

As we talked, Cleart, with a smirk on his face, said, yeah, Willis, be careful. The way you sound, Mary will have you strung out, brother. Laughing, okay, you are mimicking Stan now, but I got this under control. We were laughing as Cleart pulled into the parking lot, and we headed into the Mart Building for work.

The Intensity of Our Nightly Phone Calls
As a continuing routine, I called Mary Thursday evening at the usual time. Immediately she said, "Willis, it was nice seeing you last night. After you left, I realized you were tired, and I appreciate you coming to visit me. At first, I thought you were disappointed in seeing me."

I quickly apologized for not responding more enthusiastically when you walked into the visitors' lounge. I was exhausted from my gym workout, and that initially caused my brain to go numb momentarily. Mary, for me seeing you last night was a utopia! I had anticipated seeing you since we first met, and I am looking forward to seeing you again, very soon and often, hopefully." With emphasis, Mary said, "okay, Willis, we will have to work on getting to see one another soon, okay."

She then said, "Oh, Willis, how was your taxicab ride home last night?" I had to collect myself after hearing Mary say; we will have to work on us seeing each other again soon. I was now smiling; however, I had to tamper down my verbal response, so Mary would not detect how eager I was to see her again.

I casually responded, "My cab ride home was fine, but I practically fell asleep in the cab, and when I got home, I hit the sack and went straight to sleep."

"I really enjoyed seeing you last night, Willis. However, when you are so physically exhausted, it may not be the best situation to visit me after your gym workout. Maybe you should visit me on the weekend when I am at home," she stated.

Letting me know that "I could come to her home on the weekend to see her was cool." My ego antenna went up exponentially, and I let Mary know that would work just fine for me. We said good night, and I was now anticipating the weekend arriving in a few days.

The Courtship Visiting Mary's Home
Based on the personal vibes between Mary and me, I was convinced that she was enamored with me, the same as I admired her. She was interested enough to invite me to her home and, in effect, to meet her parents. I knew in the African-American cultural experience, a young lady would invite you to her home before she would go out on a date with you.

I borrowed my dad's car on Saturday evening and drove to East St. Louis to see Mary. It was 7:55 pm when I knocked on the door. Almost immediately, Mary opened the door, displaying her familiar illuminating smile; she said, "Hi Willis, come on in."

I stepped into the house, into the living room, and said hello to Mary; she asked me to sit on the couch. I will be right back, Willis, momma's busy, but I want her to meet you." She left the room and returned, holding her mother's arm.

I stood up when they entered the living room, and the smile on Mary's face broadened, saying proudly, "Willis, this is my mother, Mrs. Byas. Momma, this is Willis Drake, a friend from St. Louis." I moved a few steps closer to her mother, extending my right hand. I grasped her right hand with both hands and said, "hello, Mrs. Byas; I am glad to meet you."

Mrs. Byas' smile was so natural and genuine, and I felt welcomed in her home. I could see where Mary got her beautiful smile. Mrs. Byas said, "Willis, it is nice to meet you. She apologized for not having time to talk now. She was in the middle of sewing a dress that had to be finished tonight, and she left the living room."

Mary and I sat on the couch and had an interesting conversation. She whispered, "Willis, my little sisters are peeping at us, and they are laughing their hearts out. I turned my head slightly to see them amusingly looking at their big sister and me.

Mary quickly beckons for them to come into the living room. In a flash, they were standing next to their big sister, "Pookie," giggling. Mary helped them up on the couch, with Margaret Ann sitting on her right and Mona sitting on her left, between Mary and me.

With her arms around her little sisters, she said, "Willis, these are my two "big girls." This is Mona, and this little one is Margaret Ann. I said hello to them. They both, in their youthful shyness, said hi. Mary's brothers came into the living room, and she said these are my brothers, David, and Terry. They said a quick hi and left the room as quickly as they had appeared.

Mary said to her sisters, "you have met Willis; now you can go play, okay." Reacting on cue, Mona and Margaret Ann scooted down from the couch, giggling as they ran from the living room. Mrs. Byas hollered, "Mona and Margaret Ann, stop running before you fall and break your neck."

I had met Mary's mother, brothers, and sisters, and I felt comfortable at her home. Now we were alone, laughing, talking, and enjoying ourselves. Neither Mary nor I were very talkative, but we seemed to talk more when we were together. The first time I visited Mary at the Homer G. Phillips dormitory, we talked continuously, just as we had done when we first met.

Throughout the evening, our interactions allow us to discuss some idiosyncrasies and enjoy our small talk. We were intermittently touching hands, flirting, and having a good time together. Mary's personality and mannerisms profoundly struck me as we interacted during the evening.

Inconspicuously, I was also feasting my eyes on how fine Mary looked. After all, her physical attributes were the immediate attention that initially caught my eye. Tonight she was wearing dark blue slacks and a light bluish blouse, and her hair was "together." She looked the way that I remembered her the first time we met.

Close to an hour had passed when we heard a key in the front door. Mary said with a smile, "That's my dad," as she got up to open the door for him. She said, "hi, dad," as he came into the house with a White Castle bag in each hand.

I stood up as Mary's father was now in the living room. He smiled and said hi, Pookie, and his eyes focused on me. Mary guided her dad closer to the couch and said, "Daddy, I want you to meet Willis Drake, a friend from St. Louis." I extended my hand and said hello, Mr. Byas; I am pleased to meet you, sir. He shifted the White Castle bag from his right hand, and we shook hands. He said, "hello, young man; it's nice to meet you, Willis."

Hearing their father's voice, Mona and Margaret Ann came running into the living room. Mrs. Byas' voice echoed in the background, "stop that running." As the girls reached the living room, Mr. Byas bent down and hugged his baby girls. They blurted out, "Hi, daddy," and Mona and Margaret Ann, now with the White Castle bags, headed to the kitchen. Mr. Byas followed his baby girls.

Now alone in the living room, Mary said, "Daddy brings White Castles hamburgers home on Saturdays, but I very seldom eat any. I like the White Castle fish sandwich, and I will eat them sometimes."

As we continued talking, it was obvious that Mary was pleased that I had met her father too. Mary said, "my dad is very nice, but he is quiet until he gets to know you. However, momma is more talkative and will ask you questions about anything on her mind." We both laughed, and I confirmed that sounds like my parents' personality-wise, as well.

We talked for several hours that evening, and I told Mary what a wonderful time I had, but I didn't want to stay too late. In her soft voice, she said, "Willis, I am glad you came, and I really enjoyed spending this evening with you. However, "It's just 10:30, and it is okay to stay until 11:00 o'clock."

I quickly thought about the idea and decided I didn't want to overstay my first visit to her home. Mary fully understood the situation, and as I was ready to leave, I asked if I could say goodnight to her parents.

Smiling, she took my hand, and we went to the kitchen doorway, and I said goodnight to her mom and dad. They both pleasantly said, "Good-night," and Mrs. Byas said, "it was nice meeting you, Willis, and be careful driving home."

Mary was in front of me as we walked from the kitchen to the front door, and we said goodnight in the living room. Driving home, I navigated driving across the Eads Bridge through downtown St. Louis, and in no time, I was at Delmar and Newstead Avenues, one block from my home.

I parked the car in front of the house, and I was feeling spry as I jogged up the front steps. I was humming a popular song as I went into the house and went straight up upstairs to my bedroom.

After the First Visit to Mary's Home

The days had now extended into weeks, with intensity, and it was now late October. We had a sparse social life, basically spending time on weekends together as we were getting to know one another better.

As young adults, Mary and I enjoyed having fun, but neither of us often frequented nightclubs or lounges for routine entertainment. As a rule, we were not alcohol drinkers. Therefore, on weekends mostly, I visited Mary's home on Saturday evenings; we would go to the movies, local dances, and out to eat, and we would just be together doing fun things.

As we dated, Mary and I never said those unique words: "Dating exclusively or going steady." There was chemistry between us that we understood, there was no one else we were interested in dating, and therefore our relationship was exclusive.

Our friendship was still in a developing stage, but in this brief time, within me, I knew it was moving fast into a meaningful relationship.

Therefore, I always found a way to get to East St. Louis to see Mary. Between using my dad's car and borrowing my friend Cody's (Norbert Cody) car, I was always able to visit her at her home.

In the middle of the week, occasionally on a Wednesday, after leaving the gym, I would stop by the HGP Dorm to see Mary. As our relationship started to sparkle, Mary felt some of her classmates were just being nosy as they inquired if we were going steady. That irritated her, particularly if the classmates were not her close friends. With a sarcastic laugh, she said, "Some of my classmates just want to get into my business."

"Willis, during our serious girl talks, some classmates mentioned that you are a nice guy and good-looking too. I told my classmates that we are seriously dating, and that meant hands off to everybody," she said.

Looking directly at me, she said, "Willis, don't let those comments go to your head, okay." I was laughing, but Mary was dead serious and not smiling; it was more of a smirk on her face. Now our laughter increased, and Mary had the last word on that.

As a freshman class, the nursing students had established a remarkable sisterhood relationship among themselves. They shared information with their classmates about mutual acquaintances and friends they knew. Also, Mary was well-liked by her classmates, and they looked out for her as she was one of the youngest student nurses at HGP.

Mary's classmates, Julia Bruce, and Ollie Carlisle (Brookings) graduated in my June 1958 Sumner High School class. Mary had excellent character references from both of them regarding me. I had known Julia since the fifth grade at Marshall Elementary school.

Starting the New Year, January 1960, Mary and I had been dating exclusively for five months. A few of Mary's classmates tried to interest her in going out with a friend or their brother, but Mary discreetly let her classmates know that she was in an exclusive relationship and that she was not available or interested in dating anyone else at this time.

Mary's Academics

As we continued cultivating our personal and romantic relationship, Mary was focused on taking care of her business in the classroom. We both understood she needed to maintain sufficient academic grades to remain eligible for the Homer G. Phillips nursing program.

Mary was candid with me regarding maintaining her grades. Routinely our dates consisted of spending time together on weekends. She understood the director of nursing, Miss. Minnie Edith T. Gore's inflexible attitude concerning a student with failing grades. She was forthright to apprise students, "Don't let the door hit you as you leave." She strived to have one of the best nursing programs in the city and the country as well.

During the regular school year, Mary was able to engage with her family on the weekends and also see me as well. We had more liberal time during her Christmas holiday school break to socialize. We would attend parties, dances, and music concerts or go to a nightclub. We basically did whatever Mary wanted to do, but the paramount factor was us spending time together.

Getting to know Mary over the five months was marvelous. In reality, I was confronted with distinguishing between impetuous passion, natural hormonal lust, and the true expression of deep feelings bordering on love.

At some point in every relationship, spoken, perceived, or demonstrated, there is a moment that defines the commitment two people make to "one another." That time, or the moment they know they truly love each other." I ascribed "The Walk" as that moment for Mary and me.

A "cliché or an aphorism" have been expressed to describe an individual's experience when they first knew "that person" was the one for them! Sentiments articulated as "when I first laid eyes on him/her it was love at first sight; or when we first kissed I heard bells ringing, and the earth moved under my feet."

My experience was completely different. "The Walk" is when I knew Mary was "the one!" It was not romantic, but it was clearly the defining moment when I knew Mary Ann Byas and I absolutely loved one another unquestionably.

"The walk" spanned a twenty-five-minute trek from Homer G. Phillips nursing dormitory to my home at 4462 Enright Avenue. The walk shaped our lives, encompassing love and happiness, and concluded with "fifty-five years of a happy marriage."

It was bone-chilling cold that evening, and metaphorically "The Hawk" was talking!" I arrived at Homer G. dormitory in a taxicab close to six o'clock that evening. I was anticipating taking Mary to my house all week to meet my mother for the first time. Surprisingly, Mary appeared in the lobby immediately after I arrived. Normally, it would take her 10 or 15 minutes to come to the lobby. Had I known she would be so punctual, I would have asked the cab driver to wait.

I asked Mary to call the Allen Taxicab Company to send a taxicab to pick us up. Normally, a taxicab would arrive in 5 minutes; however, this was Christmas week, so the taxicab service was off schedule. As usual, not as many taxicabs were in service during this Christmas week.

We waited fifteen minutes without a taxicab showing up, so Mary called the taxi dispatcher again, inquiring when the cab would arrive. The dispatcher sounded agitated by Mary's follow-up phone call. She said, "The taxis' were backed-up, and it will be an hour for a taxi to pick you up."

With my "infinite wisdom," I asked Mary if she wanted to walk two blocks and catch the Taylor bus to get to my house. Displaying her beautiful smile, she agreed to catch the bus. I was aware that young ladies normally would not ride a bus on a date, particularly in freezing weather or walking wearing high heels shoes. However, Mary was willing and said, "sure, catching the bus is fine." At that precise moment, I should have realized that Mary was exceptional.

It was extremely cold out; the temperature was nearly freezing. We left the dormitory, and the bristling wind was immediately upon our faces in a penetrating fashion. Mary was holding my arm tightly as we walked fast as we could. It only took us about seven minutes to reach the Taylor Avenue bus stop. However, after waiting five minutes, there was still no bus in sight.

Unfortunately, unbeknownst to me, the buses were running behind schedule too. Now we were outside, exposed to the wintry weather. We started walking, hand in hand, as Mary snuggled close against my right shoulder. We would catch the bus when it came to that bus stop where we were.

I lived one and a half miles from Homer G. dormitory. We were dressed for cold winter weather but not to be exposed to near-freezing temperatures for a long time. Mary was wearing a black coat and black high heel shoes, with a black and gray scarf on her head. I had on my winter coat and my Dobbs hat.

We continued walking towards my home as the wind's velocity increased. I constantly looked over my shoulder, hoping a bus would come quickly, so we could escape the blistering cold weather. We were in lockstep, walking shoulder to shoulder. With our gloves on, Mary and I held hands. With her right hand, she was tightly holding onto my arm. We were walking, talking, and being as close together physically to one another as possible.

Somehow being together, despite the cold temperature and high winds that evening, we managed to appear comfortable. In jest, the old cliché "when you are in love, you do not feel the cold, was a euphemism or an understatement in our case."

Mary's willingness to walk in this extreme weather condition instead of demanding we catch a taxicab was phenomenal. Walking with me solidified our constantly evolving and developing relationship. Since we first met, I felt that Mary cared for me, and her feeling was beyond superficial. However, the experience of "The Walk" confirmed that we cared for each other immensely!"

I also considered that Mary was wearing high-heeled shoes and did not complain during the walk. Only once did she admit to being a little cold. Then she just held onto my arm a little tighter, snuggling closer to me to stay warm. Her actions were much more than just walking in the inclement weather with me.

In the African-American culture I grew up in, it would be preposterous to think that a young African-American (black) woman would walk a mile in high heel shoes and freezing temperatures to her date's home. Even more so, riding a bus on a date was not apropos or conducive to furthering a meaningful developing or evolving relationship.

When we reached the Hodiamont bus stop, we saw the Taylor bus approaching. At that point, we were one block from where I lived. It had taken us twenty-five minutes to walk a mile and a half, from Homer G. dormitory, in the bitterly cold weather, to a block from my house on Enright Avenue.

We reached my house and rushed inside to escape the swirling cold weather that was biting to the bone. With alarm in her voice, mother called out, "who is that?" Trying to shake the chilliness from my body, I responded, "hi, mom, it's me, and Mary is with me." Her voice was calm, saying okay, Willis, for a minute, you startled me rushing in the house so fast like that."

Mary was shivering slightly, and I helped take off her coat and put our coats on the coat tree in the vestibule. I could now see Mary in her black dress and black shoes, with appropriate accessories accentuating her attire. She looked stunning, as fine as ever to me! After walking a mile and a half in high heel shoes, she did not look frazzled as if she needed to recuperate in any way.

Mary and I were standing in the family room, and mother had ended her telephone conversation, and she approached us smiling as usual. I introduced Mary to my mother, and her smile was as bright as my mother's smile.

In her usual friendly way, mother said, "Mary, it is so nice to meet you; Willis has mentioned you often." Mary responded, "It is really nice to meet you, Mrs. Drake." Mother, with her hand on Mary's arm, said, "sweetheart, have a seat here on the couch and make yourself comfortable."

In retrospect, that evening, "the walk" and visiting my home apparently proved to be very fulfilling for both Mary and I. That cold winter night in December 1959, I truly knew I loved Mary Ann Byas, and she expressed the same feelings for me.

Additionally, that evening was when my mother saw Mary in person for the first time, and unbeknownst to me, Mary was the girl that was revealed three times in my mother's vision three years earlier, in 1956, when I was 16 years old.

Mary and I had only known each other for four months, but the short time was unimportant. We had realized, without having to vocalize, that the emotional and romantic feelings we had for one another were real! Obviously, our feelings were more than a fledging fling, which can exist with teenagers. However, our feelings had grown exponentially sufficiently that they now were like a passion, being molded into the "true feelings we professed feeling for each other."

Sometimes articulation of words is not necessary for your true feelings to be manifested. That was the case with Mary and me. We were able to discern while walking a mile and a half in extremely cold weather, the true depth of our togetherness. Subsequent to the "Walk" in the following days, my confidence was sky-high. Knowing that Mary and I had genuine mutual feelings for one another was unquestionable.

Many years later, I referred to that evening as "The Walk," and it indeed boosted my self-confidence regarding the feelings (love) that Mary truly had for me.

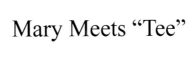

Mary Meets "Tee"

GROWING UP IN ST. LOUIS, my mother's sister Ethel Mae Sanford who her nieces and nephews called Tee, was our only aunt living in the city where we lived. My father's sisters live in Memphis, Tennessee, and we only saw them when we visited Memphis in the summertime.

Following the New Year, January 1960, Mary and I had solidified our relationship, and we were officially exclusively dating. At this point, I had made it known, especially to my sisters Shirley, Jean, and Joan, and my "boys" (Stan McKissic, Garland Greer, James Anderson, and Cleart Jones) that Mary and I were "going steady."

I only had two uncles, my father's older brothers, Uncle Alex and Uncle Oddie, who lived in a different state. I had introduced Mary to my mother during the Christmas holidays. Now I wanted to introduce Mary to my favorite aunt "Tee." Growing up, Tee was that person in our family whom her nieces and nephews would candidly discuss and confide in her about everything.

Shortly after New Year's Day, I stopped at Tee's house to wish her a Happy New Year. As we were having a routine conversation, I mentioned that I had spent Mary's entire Christmas break with her last week.

We had gone skating, to the movies, and to a nightclub in Brooklyn, IL, near East St. Louis that teenagers went to on weekends. Tee laughed, yes "Bill" (My mother's nickname) told me you brought Mary to the house to meet her last week."

Willis, I want to meet Mary! Maybe you could bring her to the house on Thursday; I am off work that day. I will fix a little snack so we can have a bite, and I can meet and talk with Mary." Willis, over all the years we have talked, I don't remember you talking about any girlfriend like you talk about Mary! I can see in your face, and hear in your voice, that you really care for her in a special way."

I acknowledged, "Yes, Tee, Mary is special to me!" I was grinning unabashedly as I left her house. When I got home, I called Mary to let her know we were invited to Tee's house Thursday evening. That she mostly just wanted to meet you. However, she will have a snack for us to eat also.

Willis, you have talked so much about Tee; I really want to meet her. Yes, Thursday evening will be fine for me." I was pleased that Mary seemed excited to meet Tee. After we hung up the phone, I immediately called Tee to let her know that Mary and I would see her Thursday at 6:00 o'clock; but Mary could only stay for about an hour.

On Thursday evening, I called Mary just before I left to pick her up. When I pulled up in front of the dorm, she quickly came out, and before I could open the car door for her, she had slid into the seat next to me. The word hello rolled off her tongue as she settled comfortably in the car. She immediately started to tell of her encounters of the day.

We arrived at Tee's house and walked up the five marble steps I was most familiar with from my childhood living in this apartment. I knocked on the door, and I told Mary, "This doorbell hasn't worked since I was a kid." Tee opened the door, and with her captivating smile, she said, "Hello, you are Mary; come on in."

We were in the hallway as we greeted Tee. She said, "Willis, please show Mary into the living room and make yourselves comfortable.

I will be with you in a minute." Mary sat on the couch, and I sat in the living room guest chair as I always did.

It was only a few minutes, and Tee had returned to the living room. Sitting next to Mary, she said, "Mary, I understand your time is limited this evening. I have wanted to meet you because my nephew has mentioned you so much. I have just a light snack, and we can talk while eating.

We went to the kitchen, where Tee had prepared tuna salad with Krispy crackers, sliced tomatoes, orange juice, and of course, Jell-O for dessert. This was Tee's standard menu when she invited her nieces and nephews over for a "confidential" talk.

We were now seated at the kitchen table, and Tee started a polite conversation with Mary. They talked about how school was going; Mary explained that she was doing well in general, but her math-based courses dealing with dispensing medications were more difficult. "Tee, I am enjoying nursing school despite the hard work," said Mary.

As Mary and Tee talked, they were laughing and seemed comfortable with one another right away. They both had pleasing and friendly personalities. Additionally, their common interest in nursing is possibly another reason they clicked so well. Tee was a Licensed Practical Nurse (LPN).

Some of the terminology and jargon I did not readily comprehend. As I finished eating my food, I observed the two women interacting like colleagues that had known one another for a short time. It boosted my confidence because I could see that Tee really liked Mary and vice versa.

I politely interrupted their conversation and reminded Mary that she had to return to the dorm shortly. Okay, but I will help Tee clean up the kitchen first. Tee said, "Mary, don't worry about washing those few dishes, kiddo. I will get them later."

Mary insisted, "Tee together; it will only take us a few minutes to wash and dry these few dishes." Over her hearty laugh, Tee said okay, kiddo, and they continued talking and cleaned the kitchen. I sensed the mutual admiration between Tee and Mary in just forty-five minutes together.

Tee gave Mary an affectionate hug as we were leaving. I hugged Tee and thanked her for everything. Joking, I said the tuna salad tasted good. Did you use something special this evening? Tee tapped me on my shoulder and said Willis, get out of here; you are a mess.

In the car, Mary said, "She enjoyed meeting and talking with Tee. Willis, one of my favorite foods is tuna salad with crackers. I often fix it when I am home on the weekends."

I laughed and said, "Mary Tee was spot-on because one thing that she was good at making was tuna salad." I pulled in front of the Homer G. dormitory and walked Mary to the lobby of the dormitory, and we said goodnight.

I returned home and went into the house. Mother was watching TV, and before I could take my coat off, she asked how everything went at Ethel's." Mother, everything went really well. I could tell that Mary and Tee seemed to click with one another, and we had a terrific evening.

Mother said, "you are right. Ethel was impressed with Mary, and she really likes her. She also thinks Mary is a very pretty girl. She said you have that Drake touch and know how to pick your girls." You know, I also think Mary is a pretty young lady, and I can tell she is smart." Smiling broadly, I agreed with mother, and we laughed.

I was buoyed by the chemistry between Tee and Mary, just meeting for the first time. I rose from the couch, kissed mother on the forehead, and went upstairs. This was the time every evening I would kick back and relax, call, and talk to Mary on the phone with the music playing on the radio in the background. I waited as the phone rang and looked forward to hearing Mary's voice on the other end.

Mary's New School Semester Year
The reality of "The Walk" had culminated, and my emotions reached another level between Mary and I. The days and weeks seemed to pass

quickly. I found myself calling Mary more often, and our telephone conversations lasted longer. My visits occurred during the week, at the nurse's dorm, and sometimes I only stayed fifteen minutes.

My feelings had grown exponentially stronger, and I wished I could see Mary more often. It was obvious that Mary also had reciprocal emotional feelings, the same as I was experiencing.

It was a mutual reaction that we were experiencing as young emotional young adults. With every look, touch, and heartbeat, that natural desire of an eighteen and nineteen-year-old male and female surfaced.

It was now apparent that after this period in our relationship, Mary and I loved one another completely. It was not just physical attraction or human passion. We knew the distinction between those emotions that were physical, hormonal, lust, or what human desires emanate. However, we both knew we cared deeply for one another and loved one another internally.

Just as the old year ended, the New Year began with Mary and I talking every night. Time seemed to fly by quickly in the New Year. Month after month, we constantly enjoyed each other's companionship. Based on Mary's schedule, we had nailed down when we could talk on the phone and when we would go out on a date.

Mary and I were now seven months into our continuing, rapidly developing, and serious relationship. The feelings caused by our emotional passion for each other had reached a point of human submission.

—◇—

CHAPTER 7

The Conversation

—◇—

MARY AND I WERE YOUNG adults, but in actuality, we were still just teenagers. We were embarking on the apex of our romantic relationship. We had dated exclusively for seven months, and the human element and natural instincts of vibrant young adults surfaced naturally.

Our emotional feelings were being challenged and put to the extreme test as we were faced with our natural vivacity, enthusiasm, and bonafide love for one another. When we were together one evening, emotionally, we were overwhelmed. On this occasion, logic, reasonableness, rational thinking, and moral restraint were supplanted by our passionate human emotions. Then extemporaneously, we had one copious emotional outburst of our human passions: an overwhelming romantic encounter we did not control. Subsequently, within a month, Mary and I had "The Conversation."

This particular Friday was dramatically different and unexpected! The phone rang, and I was surprised to hear Mary's voice. She sounded so grim, as her voice was cracking with emotion, and she said Willis, please can you come to pick me up so we can talk!

By the tone of her voice, I detected there was something "wrong." I responded immediately, with a sense of urgency, okay baby, yes; I will be there in twenty-five minutes. I looked at my watch, and it was 7:20 pm. I asked Mary if everything was okay. With her voice softer than normal, she said Willis; I just need to talk with you. When you get here, I will come out to the car.

I borrowed my dad's car and left the house posthaste, driving with urgency to the Homer G. dorm. I could not erase from my mind Mary's sound of anxiousness and maybe despair on the phone.

When I arrived at the dorm, Mary came out immediately and descended the dormitory steps; however, she did not display her swift rhythmic, bouncing motion of energy as usual. Instead, she appeared to be in slow motion coming down the steps as if the world's weight was on her shoulders.

My eyes were firmly affixed on her as she got in the car. She seemed so different in every way. Her radiant smile and vibrant normal hello were absent as she slid into the car seat. She was now sitting next to me, and absent was her normal gaiety.

Enthusiastically saying hi, baby, I softly stroked her face with my right hand and gently squeezed her left hand as I usually did. She manufactured an artificial smile and leaned over, and kissed me lightly on my lips. Her actions and motions seemed robotic. Nothing she did to this point was natural or real, as she seemed to be in a "funk" or a state of shock.

I was befuddled and being redundant; again, I asked, "Mary is everything alright?" Not looking at me, she said, "Willis, please, I just want to go someplace so we can talk!" Without saying another word, I pulled away from the dormitory. I turned left on Cottage Avenue, drove past Sumner High School, and continued driving west without a specific destination in mind. Everything seemed opaque and vague to me at this point, and the silence was deafening in the car.

I turned on the radio to our favorite R&B station, and the music was the only sound in the car. Mary had not said two words since we had been driving. However, I could perceptively tell something was pressing heavily on her mind.

Suddenly I saw the White Castle, and I realized that we were at Natural Bridge and Kingshighway Boulevards. I turned into the White Castle's parking lot and parked where few cars were, so we could talk. On Friday evenings, the White Castle was busy with young people buying the popular $0.12 hamburger, a soda, and French fries. The parking lot was busy.

I asked Mary if she wanted something to eat, in part trying to stimulate a conversation. She stared straight in front of her and just shook her head from side to side without saying anything, indicating that she did not want anything to eat.

Mary was sitting with her back halfway against the passenger door, facing me. She had an uncanny facial expression and a look of distress as if she was all alone in the world—Mary, whom I absolutely love, displayed a demeanor unseen by me before. I could not imagine what had created such an appearance of despair as she gazed into space.

I was bewildered, so I injected humor, commenting on her "fly" outfit." Hoping this would cheer her up and bring a smile to her face. Instead, her eyes were filled with tears. Then she spoke, saying softly, "Willis, I am pregnant." I paused for a few seconds making sure I heard what she said. Mary, did you say you are pregnant? Are you sure?" She repeated herself, with a slight tone of anguish in her voice. Saying emphatically, "yes, yes, Willis, I am certain!"

I was stunned to hear the word "pregnant." I was shocked, and with emphasis, "Mary, we were only intimate that one time when our emotions overwhelmed us." Through her flowing tears, she said, "yes, Willis, I know we only had sex one time, and obviously, that is when I got pregnant."

With my eyes encompassing her fragile essence, I could see the fear or possibly the sorrow in her eyes. I slid closer and drew her nearer to me, embracing her tightly. She was crying profusely now as I held her in my arms. To see her sobbing penetrated my heart, and my emotions started to swell also. Looking into her eyes, I told her, "I love you very much, and I want to marry you now."

Rhetorically, I asked, "do you love me?" She raised her head and looked straight into my eyes. Her tears had partially stopped, and with a passion in her voice, she said, "Willis, I love you so much." Her voice was so penetrating it seemed like an echo was reverberating inside the car.

Now, that beautiful smile started to emerge and appear on her face. Then in a reserved fashion, she confided that "Willis being so young, I was not sure that you wanted to get married now." With total emphasis, I again told her, "I truly love you and want you to be my wife." Mary looked very solemn, and in a subdued voice, she said; Willis, I want to finish nursing school, and I know my parents had their minds also set on me finishing school and being a nurse.

I imagine Mary's feelings were conflicted at this precise moment, knowing her parents would be disappointed. To lift her spirit, I let Mary know I would talk to her parents immediately, asking for their permission and blessings for us to get married.

However, I want them to know I love you very much, and we have decided to get married now. I also assured Mary that after we are married, I will do everything possible so she can finish nursing school.

It was now several hours later, and with emotions stretched and uncertainty staring us in our faces, we had completed "**The Conversation**." Subsequent to our impactful "conversation," I assured Mary that everything was going to be fine. If there was any fear in me, I did not show it! I demonstrated the emotional strength of a husband-to-be and that I would take care of her.

I drove from the White Castle to take Mary back to the HGP dormitory. Finally, she managed a semi-smile and snuggled close to me with her head on my shoulder. Our favorite radio station was playing soft groovy romantic R & B music, and Mary seemed calm, relaxed, and at ease now.

Arriving at the dormitory, we sat in the car talking until it was Mary's curfew time. Holding hands, we walked to the dorm's steps and again affirmed our love for one another. Ascending the steps, Mary said good night with a smile as she entered the dorm.

Driving home, my thoughts were focused on my immediate obligation to talk with Mary's parents. I wanted their permission and blessings; however, Mary and I had decided unequivocally that we would get married right away. We would not consider any other option!

I arrived home and went straight to my bedroom. So many thoughts were still swirling around in my head. I had not encountered anything of this magnitude before in my life. I turned on the radio, and as the music filtered through it, it helped clear my mind. I needed to let my parents know that Mary and I were getting married. Thirty minutes later, after digesting several scenarios, I turned off the radio and went to sleep.

I woke up Saturday morning, and instantly my thoughts focused on Mary and how she was feeling this morning. It was noon time when I called her, and we continued our conversation from last night. We both again reaffirmed that we were totally committed to getting married next month.

We decided that I would pick Mary up Tuesday evening after her last class, and we would drive to East St. Louis so I could let her parents know we were going to get married. Subsequently, I would also tell my parents about our plans.

Talk With Mary's Parents
The emotional conversations Mary and I had over the weekend caused the time to fly by so quickly. Now we were in our normal routine, and Monday night Mary and I talked much longer than usual. I never detected any reservation, doubt, or concern in Mary's conversation or attitude

regarding us getting married. Apparently, she was clear in our decision to get married the next month, the same as I was.

Before hanging up the phone, I reminded Mary that I would pick her up at 5:30 pm tomorrow. "Okay," she said confidently, "I will be in the lobby waiting when you get here," and we said good night.

I could not go to sleep right away. I was preoccupied with thoughts of how and what I would say to Mary's parents. I tossed and turned until I was exhausted, and finally, at 3:00 am, I went to sleep. In the morning, I got ready as usual and went to work.

By midday, I felt physically and mentally rejuvenated. When I got home from work that evening, I still had not conceptualized in my mind how and what I would say to Mary's parents. I went into the house and quickly went upstairs and changed my clothes. Returning downstairs, I went to the kitchen, said hello to mother, and told her I was going to see Mary. (I did not mention that I was going to East St. Louis to talk with Mary's parents).

I had arranged to use my dad's car, and he had left the car key on the mantelpiece in the family room. I grabbed the car key and rushed out of the house. As planned, I had about 25 minutes to pick up Mary at 5:30 pm.

The traffic was light driving to get Mary. I pulled up in front of the nurses' dormitory, and she was waiting at the entrance. It was 5:25 pm, and she quickly came down the steps and got in the car. Mary leaned over, kissed me, and said, "I love you, Willis Drake." She appeared upbeat, considering we were going to tell her parents, without their prior knowledge, that we were getting married.

I responded to Mary's routine affection in a suave manner, saying, "I love you too, Mary Byas," as I drove from the dormitory. Strangely enough, I will always remember this day. It was early March 1960. I was driving to East St. Louis, Illinois, with Mary by my side to ask her parents for their permission and blessings to marry their daughter, Mary Ann Byas (aka Pookie).

Driving to Mary's Home:
Over the past months, I had driven to Mary's home numerous times. It would take thirty-five minutes to drive from Homer G. to Mary's house at 919 11th Street in East St. Louis. After crossing over the Mississippi River, on the Eads Bridge, it would only take five minutes to get to her house.

As we were driving, I could sense perhaps that Mary was somewhat preoccupied. Her parents would be unprepared (blindsided) by me seeking their approval to marry Mary now. Given the circumstance, her parents would be disappointed and likely concerned for Mary's future. In reality, we were just 18 and 19-year-old teenagers planning to get married.

I had always felt comfortable talking to Mary's parents, and despite the situation, I hoped it would be the same this evening. I was trusting in Lord God Almighty and knowing everything would be all right. I still did not know the words I would say to Mary's parents.

I parked the car in front of Mary's house, and we looked at each other for a minute, and I asked, "are you ready?" She smiled, and we got out of the car and walked to the front door holding hands. With her door key in hand, Mary fumbled for a few seconds trying to open the door. Joking, I asked, "Are you nervous, baby?" Smiling, she said, "I must be nervous if I cannot open my front door."

We entered the house and were in the living room when Mrs. Byas came into the room. The look on her face let me know she was surprised to see us. She said, "Pookie, I heard the front door open, and it startled me." She hugged Mary and said, "hi Willis, how are you this evening? "Hello, Mrs. Byas; I am doing fine," I responded.

With her natural smile adorning her face, she said, "Pookie, I did not know you were coming home this evening, is everything okay?" Mary said, "Momma, Willis wants to talk to you and daddy." Mrs. Byas' eyes were now focused on me. Without hesitation, I said, Mrs. Byas, I would like to speak with you and Mr. Byas if I can.

With a puzzled look, Mrs. Byas said, "Pookie, your father is in the back room." Apparently, hearing Mary's voice, Mr. Byas walked into the living room. He said hello to Mary and I, and we exchanged our hello greetings. As she moved towards the couch, Mrs. Byas said, "Matt Byas, Willis wants to talk with us."

Mary's parents were now sitting on the couch. Mary was sitting in the living room chair across the room from the couch, and I was standing next to her. We were facing her parents, and I immediately said, "Mr. and Mrs. Byas, I love Mary very, very much; and she loves me too." I am asking for your permission and blessings to marry Mary next month.

Mrs. Byas' facial and Mr. Byas' stoic expressions revealed that they were totally caught off guard by my request. Having quickly gathered her composure, Mrs. Byas said, "Willis, what about Mary's nursing school? Matt Byas and I want her to finish nursing school before she gets married.

Why don't you just wait until she finishes school?" Standing next to Mary, I wasn't exactly sure how to say it. Then unconsciously, the words came out of my mouth. "Mary is pregnant, and I want to marry her now."

There was a short period of silence, and looking at us, Mr. Byas, in a disturbed voice, said, "Pookie is this what you want to do?" Mrs. Byas interrupted at that point and said, "Pookie, Matt Byas and I have to talk. You go back to school and call me when you get there so we can talk." They got up from the couch, and Mrs. Byas' demeanor reflected disappointment, and Mr. Byas' reaction was the same.

As we were leaving the house, Mary's mom hugged her. Then she said, "Willis, drive safely going back to St. Louis, and Matt Byas and I will talk with you tomorrow." I assured them that I would drive carefully.

Driving Back to Homer G. Phillips

Notwithstanding our situation and the fact that her parents said they would talk with me tomorrow, I felt comfortable having officially asked for their permission and blessings to marry Mary next month.

We were at Mary's house for only fifteen or twenty minutes, and now it was past twilight, and we were driving across the Eads Bridge, returning to Homer G. dormitory. I felt assured that Mary and I would get married with her parents' permission and blessings.

I turned on the radio, and the Dee Jay was locked into playing the music and songs that was so apropos of what we needed to hear now. Mary turned the radio volume up as she scooted closer and nestled her head on my shoulder.

She said, "Willis, I know it will be tough, but I still want to finish nursing school after we are married. "Mary, with every breath within me, I will do everything possible so you will finish nursing school."

We were now parked in front of the dorm. We sat and listened to our favorite song as it came to an end, with the rhythmic high and low sounds fluctuating in the car. I turned off the car's engine and walked Mary to the dormitory entrance. In a fleeting moment, we said good night as I told her again, "I love you very much, Mary Byas."

I felt happy seeing her beautiful smile return on her face as she entered the dormitory. I knew she would have an emotional telephone conversation with her parents shortly. However, I knew everything would be alright.

Driving home, I had a calm and relaxed feeling about everything. The feeling that suddenly came over me was unexplainable. It was like something from within my inter-spirit letting me know everything would be fine.

Telling My Parents Mary and I Are Getting Married
Approaching home, I knew it was now the perfect time to tell my mom and dad that Mary and I would be getting married next month. I parked the car, and that same feeling of calmness remained with me.

I had a special "hop in my step entering the house, and I went straight to the kitchen. My dad was a staunch coffee drinker; sure enough, my mom and dad were sitting in their usual chairs at the opposite ends of the kitchen table, talking. Mother sometimes sat at the kitchen table with dad while he had his cup of coffee before he went to work.

Standing next to the kitchen table, I said, "dad, before you leave for work, I have something I want to tell you and mom." He looked up at me and said, "sit down, Willis; what's on your mind, son?

His distinct, unique half-smile was now on his face. I assumed he perceived what I wanted to tell them was important. I sat down, looking at both of them, glancing from one to the other. My mother's facial expression was of motherly concern, as her natural smile was absent.

Whenever I talked about serious matters with them, I never hesitated or beat around the bush. I immediately divulged straight out. Mom and dad, you know my girlfriend Mary; she and I have been dating seriously for seven months now. We love each other, and we are going to get married next month.

My dad was a man of few words, and regardless of what he was thinking or talking about, he seldom showed any emotional facial expressions. He was even-tempered, levelheaded, and very "wise."

Having heard my declaration of getting married, he took another sip of coffee and deliberately set the coffee cup down. He had a piercing look in his eyes, which reflected more of an inquisitive concern, and said, "Son, do you think Mary is ready to get married now? I thought her focus was finishing nursing school."

Mother was reserved, without comment at this point, allowing my dad's response to be prevailing. Then she said, "Willis, what's really going on that you and Mary want to get married next month?"

With a rapid response, "Mother, Mary is pregnant, and we are getting married now. There was a moment of silence, and then dad said, "Willis, regardless of the situation, have you asked Mary's parents for their permission to marry her?"

Yes, sir, Mary and I talked with her parents tonight, and I asked for their permission and blessing for us to get married. However, it was unexpected to them, just like it is to you and mother now. Mary's parents will talk with me again tomorrow, and I am confident they will give me their permission to marry Mary.

Now, it was time for dad to go to work. He rose from his kitchen chair and put on his jacket to leave for work. I was partially joking when I asked if he had any advice for me. He said, in a matter-of-fact way, with the same unemotional expression on his face. "Son, set a pace that you can handle," as he left for work.

Now, mother and I were in the family room, sitting on the couch, and she was looking directly into my eyes. She said, "I know you and Mary love one another. However, I know that marriage will not be easy either. Willis, you, and Mary are still young "kids." Just be sure you keep God in your lives, and your marriage will be fine."

Mother said, "The important thing is for the two of you to stay committed to each other. Most of all is to trust in the Lord God Almighty for everything, no matter what." Mother was optimistic about everything, and I attributed that to her faith in God. She believed that if you live right, "He" will take care of your needs. I also share that belief.

Mother and I continued talking about life in general and what Mary and I would be confronted with in our young marriage. Then she said, "When I have seen you and Mary together, I could tell from how she looked at you that she loves you. I also know you love her. Willis, I think you know I genuinely liked her from the first time I met Mary."

"Son, I know you and Mary will have a blessed marriage, and you will be a good husband, and she will be a good wife. I also know you will love, respect, and treat Mary right."

At this point, my mother had not made known to me that Mary was the "light brown-skinned girl" in the vision that the Holy Spirit had revealed to her when I was sixteen years old. Mother, however, recognized Mary as the perfect likeness to the girl in her vision who was going to be my wife.

Mr. and Mrs. Byas' Permission

The next evening Mary and I talked extensively on the phone. She described her conversation with her parents after returning to the dormitory last night. Her parents were very understanding. She and her mother mostly talked, and her mother wanted to make sure, regardless of my situation, that I wanted to marry you!

"Willis, my dad, will talk with you when he's home from work tonight. I know they will give their permission for us to get married. They know this is what we want to do. Willis, with the date we have in mind, you know we only have a few weeks to plan our wedding; and Momma will help plan the wedding," she said.

Our Parents Talked

That weekend I was at Mary's home, and Mrs. Byas said, "Willis, your mother called me yesterday and said, 'It was put on her heart to talk with me.'" With surprise, I looked at Mary, and I could see the suspense on her face as well.

"Your mother and I had a lengthy conversation about you and Pookie getting married, and I told Matt Byas what we talked about," she continued. My facial expression possibly revealed my total surprise that our mothers had talked. However, I knew that was the type of person my mother was. She would reach out to Mrs. Byas to offer her support during a situation like this.

Mrs. Byas was very deliberate in choosing her words. "Willis, we talked mostly about the type of young people you and Pookie are. As parents, we are both concerned that being so young, if you are really ready for marriage. Neither of us wants you to mess up your lives at such a young age.

Willis, your mother told me from an incredibly early age you have always been a very responsible person all your life. I described the type of person Pookie has always been too. I felt better after talking with your mother about you and Pookie getting married when we hung up the telephone."

Mrs. Byas, looking at Mary and said, "Pookie, Mrs. Drake said she knows you are a fine young woman, and when she first met you, she liked you immediately. Also, you would be welcomed into her family and accepted the same as one of her daughters when you are married."

Mrs. Byas' eyes now shifted to me, and she continued, "Willis, your mother also said that you will be a good husband and father, and you will always take care of Pookie and your family."

Mr. Byas normally did not talk much. At this point, he interrupted Mrs. Byas and said, Willis, you know that Pookie's mother and I wanted her to finish nursing school before she gets married. That was our hope and desire.

However, you came to us as a man, asking our permission and blessing to marry Pookie. So you have our blessings for you'll to get married. I pray that God will also bless your marriage and your family."

Before Mary and I left her house, I shook Mr. Byas' hand again. I also promised to do whatever it takes for Mary to finish nursing school. I told him I would always love and care for his daughter, Mary (Pookie).

CHAPTER 8

Parents Blessings

ONSIDERING OUR SITUATION, RECEIVING OUR parents' blessings to get married was paramount for Mary and I, but it was not mandatory. It is exhilarating for us to know that our mothers had that compelling conversation about us. Now we could focus on the practical necessities of getting married.

Driving Mary back to the dormitory, with the utmost confidence, I said, "Mary, everything is going to work out fine." Looking at me, she uttered softly, "yes, I know we will clear any hurdle for us to get married next month. Willis, we will have a small and beautiful wedding."

After leaving Mary's house, she was calm, naming what we needed to do to get married. Willis, first, we need to get my engagement and wedding rings and set our wedding date! Glancing at her, I saw a smile on her face as she continued talking, emphasizing getting her rings.

Arriving at the Homer G. dorm, Mary kissed me goodnight and exited the car." I watched as she went into the dorm. I sensed the weight she must have felt that was saddled on her shoulders. As a student, this onerous responsibility of planning a wedding was heavy. I said a silent prayer, knowing that Mary would soon be my wife and everything would be alright.

Heading home, my thoughts vacillated in my mind. Suddenly I was home, and I paused for just a few seconds and sat in the car to gather my thoughts. I had pep in my steps approaching the house, and I was happy as I opened the front door.

Mother was sitting in her usual place on the couch, and I sat next to her, hugged her, and thanked her. I explained that Mrs. Byas had told Mary and me about the long telephone conversation the two of you had regarding us. After you had talked, she knew that everything with Mary and I getting married would be fine. Mother, with her beautiful smile, said, "Willis, son, I know God will also bless you and Mary and your marriage."

The Wedding Plans

Mother, this weekend, I will let our family know that Mary and I are getting married on April 15th, Good Friday. Now with a sense of levity, I told mother that Mary's number one priority is buying her engagement and wedding rings. Mother smiled. "I totally agree with Mary. She wants that ring on her finger to let everyone know she's engaged to get married," she responded.

Yes, I understand, and we will go shopping on Tuesday to get her rings. With a strong sigh, I said, "mother, with Mary being in school all week, I have concerns that we can get everything done in time to get married next month.

Just having a small wedding with basically family members; still requires that everything falls in place timely for us to get married next month. Mother and I talked for a bit longer, and my spirit was uplifted tremendously when we finished talking.

I went upstairs and called Mary. I told her my mother suggested we get married in our home if that would be acceptable to her. She said, "Yes, Willis, your mother's home is lovely; it will be wonderful to get married there." I could tell by the sound of her voice that she was pleased with the idea.

We talked much longer than usual, and the extent of our conversation was identifying the specifics for us to get married. Getting Mary's rings was a top priority, and Mary also had to get her wedding dress. We had to apply for our marriage license and make plans for a modest wedding reception.

As we were ending our conversation, Mary said, "Willis, I know we are going to have a beautiful wedding; you just wait and see!" The joy in her voice revealed that she was happy. Like clockwork, everything was falling into place very smoothly. With a sense of accomplishment, we said goodnight and hung up the phone.

I slept well and woke up totally refreshed. I got up early, energized, and ready for the workday. I showered, and as I was getting dressed, my thoughts automatically reflected on Mary. I wondered if she had also slept well. I know her mind was at rest, knowing that things were falling into place for us to get married.

That morning I had a new gait to my walk, and my stride showed confidence in each step. I caught the bus on time with a bright outlook starting off my workday.

Mary's Wedding Rings
After work, I went to Homer G.'s dorm to pick up Mary. She was ready when I drove up and quickly got in the car. I was happy to see her so exuberant and full of life again as we were going to purchase her wedding rings.

There were two popular jewelry stores in downtown St. Louis that young people patronized. It was getting late, and we didn't have time to procrastinate if we wanted to get downtown before the stores closed. I didn't have a clue about buying jewelry and not engagement and wedding rings particularly.

Mary's expertise was also limited in purchasing expensive jewelry at this young age. However, she had the prerogative to select the rings she preferred based on if they appealed to her and were within our budget range.

Holding hands, like young people in love, we entered the jewelry store and were greeted by the salesperson. He was a middle-aged man, and he greeted us and immediately directed us to ring sets that were more expensive than we could afford. If that was his sales approach, to show us the most expensive rings first, it was a very poor concept.

Mary clutching my arm tightly, said, "Willis, I want to look at the rings in this showcase; it will give me an idea of different ring styles. Okay, Willis, I don't see what I want here; let's go to the other jewelry store before its closes."

The next jewelry store was on the same block. We confidently entered the store; Mary now had a better idea of the wedding ring set she liked. In a lighthearted manner, I said, "As long as we keep our eyes on the price tag, everything will be fine." Mary squeezed and pinched my hand as we started laughing like giddy teenagers.

A salesman approached us, and I explained that we were looking for a quality wedding ring set within our price range. Mary and I had agreed earlier that we did not want to start our marriage out with unreasonable financial debt.

The salesperson directed us to a showcase that had attractive wedding ring sets. They were similar to those we had seen at the previous store but were more reasonably priced. Mary meticulously looked at the rings, and when the salesman showed us the fourth set, Mary's eyes brightened considerably, and she said, "Willis, this is the ring set that I want!"

I glanced at the price tag as Mary tried the rings on to see how they fit, and they looked great on her finger. She turned to me, accentuating her pretty smile, and said, "Willis, this is the wedding ring set that I like." The rings were modest but attractive.

The rings were priced slightly above our budget range. However, I negotiated the price with the salesman, and I was able to stretch our budget a little too, and I purchased the rings. I felt satisfied knowing Mary was happy with her wedding rings.

We returned to the car, and I officially proposed to Mary. I took the engagement ring from the box and placed it on her finger, and we kissed. We arrived back at the nurses' dormitory, and we said good night. Mary bounced up the dorm's steps energetically and disappeared, getting on the elevator.

Mary called me later that night, "Willis, when I got back to the dorm, I couldn't resist showing off my engagement ring to my close friends. They were supportive of me, and they want to attend our wedding."

Hearing the joy in Mary's voice, I was delighted that she was feeling upbeat and looking forward to our wedding. Step by step, and considering everything involved, every piece of the puzzle was falling into place for us.

Mary's Wedding Gown
A few days later, Mary was extremely excited. She proceeded to tell me, "momma had gotten my wedding gown, and Willis, it is beautiful." Mary's "Wedding Gown" was borrowed from her mother's close friend who lived in St. Louis. Her friend had gotten married in her wedding gown years earlier, and it was preserved in pristine condition.

Mary and I were blessed with good fortune as our wedding plans were coming together magnificently. We now had the wedding rings, wedding gown, and the place for our nuptials next month. Listening to Mary, I was caught up in her excitement, and I said, "Mary, you will be the most beautiful bride ever." We had an extensive conversation, discussing plans before we said goodnight.

Reverend Amos Ryce II
Mary and I had an appointment to talk with my pastor Reverend Amos Ryce II, who had been my pastor for five years at the church where I was raised since I was in kindergarten. In 1954 Reverend Ryce was appointed the pastor at Lane Tabernacle Christian Methodist Episcopal (CME) Church located at 910 N. Newstead Avenue, St. Louis.

We met with Reverend Ryce on Thursday evening after Mary's last class. He asked several times, "Willis and Mary are you certain you want to get married now?" We answered unequivocally, "Yes, sir Rev. Ryce" we are going to get married on April 15th, Good Friday, at 6:00 pm at my mother's home." "Okay, I will perform your marriage ceremony," he concluded.

The Marriage License:
In the state of Missouri, for a male under the age of 21 years old to get married, he needed his parent's consent. I was only nineteen years old. However, Mary was eighteen years old, and a female 18 years old did not need her parent's consent to get married in Missouri.

Mary and I had to apply in person for our marriage license at the St. Louis City Marriage License Bureau office downtown St. Louis City Hall. My mother had to give her consent for me to get married. Thursday at 4:30 pm, my mother went with Mary and me to apply for our marriage license.

We arrived at City Hall, and I found a parking space close to the building. It was approaching closing time, and we hurried to Suite 127, where the St. Louis Marriage License Bureau was located. There was one person in line ahead of us when we arrived.

Within five minutes, Mary and I filled out the marriage license application, and mother signed, giving her consent for me to get married. The clerk informed us that the marriage license would be mailed to us within seven days.

Mary and I were satisfied to have another task completed for us to get married. I thanked mother again for coming with us to get our marriage license. Mother started laughing and said I enjoyed the ride downtown. Getting away from the house and the grandkids for a little while is refreshing. Mary and I understood the humor in mother's comment, as she babysits three or four of her grandchildren every day.

As they approached the car, Mary asked mother if she wanted to sit up front in the car. Mother looked directly into Mary's eyes and was not smiling as usual. "Mary, baby, when you're riding in the car with your husband, you always sit in the front seat, okay?

I know you are deferring to me, and I appreciate your consideration; but don't let another woman sit up front with your husband, with you riding in the backseat," mother said. Mary smiled and said, "Yes, mam, I understand."

I took mother home first, so she could have dinner before it got too late. Mary and mother said bye. I walked mother to the front door and kissed her as she went into the house. Driving back to the dorm, we were laughing, and Mary said, "one thing I will not forget though, and you better not forget it either, Willis. I won't be sitting in our car's back seat with another woman in the front seat." Mary and I both cracked up laughing.

CHAPTER 9

⬦

Mrs. Ruby Byas' Sisters

⬦

ALL WEEK AT SCHOOL, MARY was wearing her engagement ring. She was anticipating going home on the weekend, so she could show her mother her ring. Friday night Mary and I were talking on the phone, and she said, "Willis, when I came home today, momma was sitting at the kitchen table.

I walked into the kitchen and said hello to momma, as usual, placing my left hand on the kitchen table in front of her. She said, 'Pookie, when did you get your engagement ring? It's beautiful!' She hugged me, and I knew the ring represented that I was officially engaged to marry you."

"Momma was excited, admiring my engagement ring. Then she said, 'Pookie, your Aunt Mary has invited Biddy, Frances, and me to her house Sunday afternoon so you can introduce Willis to your family." Mary's voice had an element of uncertainty when she asked, "Willis, can you come on Sunday at 2:30 to meet my aunts? "Sure, that will work fine for me, and I look forward to meeting your aunts, I responded."

Terrific, and she proceeded to give me a synopsis of her aunts and their personalities. I could hear the joy in her voice. "Aunt Mary is hilarious, and you will like her," she said, and shortly after we stopped laughing, we said good night.

Mary's mother had three sisters living in the East St. Louis and St. Louis areas. Mary Ida Tolden (Aunt Mary) was the oldest sister, and the two younger sisters were Mildred Thomas (Aunt Biddy) and Frances Anderson (Aunt Frances).

Sunday afternoon, I was now driving to Mary's house; it was 2:15 pm when I arrived at her home. Mary, her mother, and sisters, Mona, and Margaret Ann, were ready to go when I got there. Mary suggested we ride in my car to Aunt Mary's and Uncle Maurice's house.

They lived at 521 Converse Street, only fifteen minutes from Mary's house. I pulled up in front of Aunt Mary's house and parked the car. Mary's young girl cousins, between five to eight or nine years old, were in front of the house expecting their cousin Pookie!

Particularly in most African-American families, traditionally or historically, there is a hierarchy structure, real or perceived, where deference is given to the oldest sibling. Mary's mother's family also adhered to this practice among the siblings.

Her Aunt Mary was the accepted, or possibly the de facto authority having the most influence among the sisters. The reality was if you received "acceptance" from Aunt Mary, it was tantamount to receiving the "stamp of approval" from Mary's mother's entire family.

We entered the house, and I stood next to Mary inside the doorway. The young cousins and Mary's aunts had coalesced inside the living room. Mary cheerfully greeted her aunts, hugging each of them. Observing as they greeted one another, it was obvious to me that Mary's family were affectionate and pleasant to be around.

Mary's family naturally wanted to meet me, the anticipated new family member who was marrying a favorite niece. Her young cousins were now sitting on the floor in the living room, taking everything in were Barbara Ann, Linda, Jo Jo (Aedella), and Renee.

They were wide-eyed, whispering and giggling amongst themselves. Young as they were, I was unsure how much they could comprehend. Their curiosity was intense, and in their minds, they wanted to meet cousin "Pookie's fiancé," who she was going to marry very soon.

Mary had her engagement ring on her finger. She wanted to officially announce to her family members, particularly her aunts, that she was engaged to marry me. I did not have any apprehension about meeting Mary's family. I imagined that it was inconceivable that Mary's character and upbringing would be unique, as opposed to being consistent with what was normal within her immediate and extended family's behavior.

Other than Mary's mom, dad, and siblings, the only other family member I had met was her Aunt, Biddy. Mary and her Aunt, Biddy, had a close aunt-and-niece relationship. Standing by Mary's side, I felt comfortable.

However, I did not know what to expect from meeting Mary's Aunt, Mary, and Aunt Frances. Entering Aunt Mary's house, the first room you walked into was the living room. The first time I crossed the threshold of her living room, she just made me feel welcome. She was a very engaging person.

With a smile on her face, Aunt Mary set the tone overall in greeting me. She was sitting in her favorite chair in the corner of the living room opposite the front door. When Mary and I walked into the house, Aunt Mary had a clear view of anyone that came into her living room. I noticed her immediately as I walked through her front door.

She was leaning forward in her chair instead of being in a reclining relaxing position. She had that illuminating smile on her face; without really knowing her, she looked like she was perched in a talking position.

Physically, Aunt Mary was a lady of short stature; likely, she was not more than five feet tall. She was a large, heavyset woman. She had the most God-given beautiful smile; and the warmest personality of almost anyone I can remember. Her human spirit was affectionate, and she was a spiritual and Christian woman.

After Mary had greeted her aunts, Mrs. Byas said, "Pookie introduce Willis to everybody." Mary, smiling, said, "okay;" she was standing close to me as she locked her right arm into my left arm. Then, with her left hand, she purposely flashed her engagement ring for everybody to see.

She said proudly, "this is my fiancé, Willis Drake. He lives in St. Louis, and we have been dating since I started nursing school last year, and we are engaged to be married." Following the introduction, Aunt Mary said, "Willis, come give your aunt Mary a hug." There were polite and happy greetings from all the family members, and I received genuine hugs from Mary's aunts. I felt warm in the crowded living room among Mary's aunts and young cousins.

Initially, the conversation was focused on me, and it was evident that Aunt Mary really enjoyed talking. She was on a roll that afternoon, and she had everyone cracking up, laughing, and having an enjoyable time. Aunt Mary's jovial and warm personality was the perfect icebreaker, and everyone was just relaxed.

Again, Aunt Mary was hovering over the conversations like a mediator. Just in case the questions from any of the aunts seemed to get more into an interrogation. With that big beautiful smile, Aunt Mary would inject something to soften the atmospheric tone.

Then with her good humor, Mary cleverly changed the conversation smoothly to reflect on her aunts. She said, Willis, Aunt Mary is the oldest sister, and she keeps everyone in line, including momma. Everybody, the aunts, and nieces, laughed at Mary's comment.

At the same time, this conversation served as a point of affirmation that Aunt Mary had the respect of her siblings. I was also laughing, but I was observing Mary, Aunt Biddy, Aunt Frances, and also Mrs. Byas.

All three of the sisters seemed to acknowledge that their big sister, Aunt Mary was the family matriarch.

In the appropriate pecking order, Aunt Mary spoke first. She said with that illuminating smile on her face. "Pookie, you have a good eye, young lady. Willis is a fine handsome young man." There was a roar, and the living room was filled with laughter, especially from Mary's young cousins. I was half-embarrassed and just smiled.

Quickly my thoughts reverted to my Aunt Tee's comment after she had met Mary for the first time. Tee told my mother, "I (Willis) surely knew how to pick my girls and that Mary was a pretty young woman."

Within the first ten minutes in Aunt Mary's living room, I could tell that Mary's aunts were alright, regular people. As it turned out, that first meeting I had with her family provided a connection that established the foundation that resulted in total and mutual endearment among me and Mary's family.

Immediately I had a warm affection for Aunt Mary, and I felt the feeling was mutual as well. I do not recall exactly how the subject came up, but the question of how I should address Mary's aunts was discussed.

With that magical personality, Aunt Mary said, "Willis, I want you to call me Aunt Mary. I already feel like you are part of our family." Then Mary's Aunt Biddy and Aunt Frances asked that I call them aunt, the same as Pookie does. I said how welcome they made me feel, and I will be pleased and comfortable calling you aunt. I could tell they truly adored their niece, Pookie.

We visited Aunt Mary's home for three hours that Sunday, which paved the way for me to have a meaningful relationship with Mary's family throughout our marriage. Upon being introduced to Mary's family, I was accepted by her family immediately, the same as my family accepted Mary.

Aunt Biddy worked as a beautician at a second, part-time job in her close friend Sarah C. Jones' Paramount Beauty Salon. The Beauty Shop Ms. Jones owned was located at 2901 N. Vandeventer Avenue, St. Louis, MO.

When Mary and I were first dating, every two weeks, Aunt Biddy would style/fix Mary's hair. Occasionally, I would pick Mary up at the beauty shop. When I walked into the shop, Aunt Biddy and Ms. Sarah would tease me, saying, "Willis, you are right on time."

I just finished tightening up Pookie's "fro," and doesn't she look good?" Smiling, I assured them that "yes, she looks beautiful." They both would burst out laughing, and Ms. Sarah said, "Willis, watch out now; as good as Pookie is looking, those young brothers out there will be checking her out big time."

Mary hugged Aunt Biddy and Ms. Sarah as we were leaving the beauty shop. Then, with a big grin, she turned and said, "Willis doesn't have to worry about my eyes wandering too far from his direction." Aunt Biddy and Ms. Sarah were laughing as we left the beauty shop.

Driving back to the dormitory, Mary said, "Willis, I hope you don't mind Aunt Biddy teasing you. She constantly reminds me to come to the shop and get my hair done every two weeks. She stresses that it is important for me to look professional, well-groomed, and pretty all the time." Laughing, I let Mary know that I understand Aunt Biddy and Ms. Sarah are joking with me, and I think you always look pretty.

After I had met Mary's mother's family a short time later, she introduced me to her father's family. Her father was the oldest son, and her uncle, Sterling, was the second oldest brother living in the East St. Louis area with his wife, Aunt Margaret.

Mary's uncle, Flarzell, was the youngest brother and his wife, Aunt Alleen; I recall meeting their daughter Corliss at that time. However, there was Wynell, Michelle, and Marva, and they also had two sons, Flarzell Jr. and Shawn Byas.

Meeting Mary's family was the last family-wise commitment that Mary and I had to address before we completed the concrete plans for our wedding.

CHAPTER 10

Mary's Desire To Be A Nurse

METAPHORICALLY SPEAKING, THE TRAIN WAS moving full steam ahead. Mary was focusing on school, so most of the wedding arrangements were being addressed by Mrs. Byas, mother, and me. Mary didn't need any obstacles to deal with regarding her classes; therefore, she stayed focused on finishing her school year in an exemplary fashion.

I understood that dreams and hopes like those Mary had may temporarily dissipate, but they do not evaporate because of one unplanned event that happened in her life. I was in total lockstep with Mary. We were of one mind and spirit to make Mary's dream a reality. Mary's ambition and desire to be a nurse was neither a whim nor a fleeting impulse.

When we had "The Conversation," and I asked Mary to marry me, I promised her that I would do everything possible for her to finish nursing school. Mary had spent nine months at the Homer G. dormitory and hospital, training and honing her skills to be a registered nurse. Encapsulated during that time was the fun she had in the dormitory, the long late-night studying, and the heart-wrenching experience of losing a young patient she was caring for in the hospital.

The memories created during those nine months were fixed in her memory alone with the image and picture of the Homer G. Phillips nurse's dormitory.

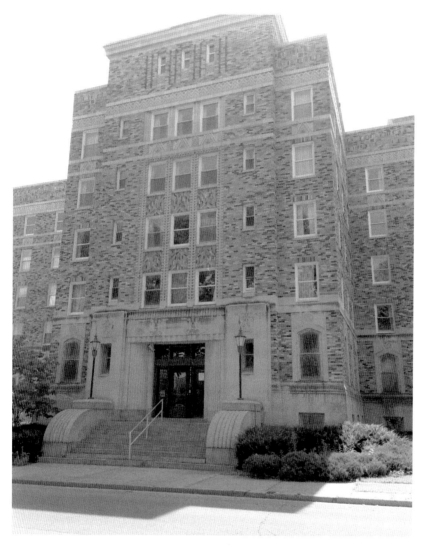

Homer G. Phillips Nurses Dormitory (2516 Goode Avenue)
https://www.bing.com/images

Unprecedented Situation—Mary's Desire To Be A Nurse:
To this day, I am not certain what allowed Mary to continue as a student nurse at Homer G. after we were married. To my understanding, there was a policy at that time (written or perceived) that a student nurse could not be married and attend the Homer G. Nursing School.

I don't know if Mrs. Byas, Mary's mother, had spoken to Miss. Gore, the Director of Nursing at that time, before Mary and I were married. I know for a fact that after Mrs. Byas talked with Miss. Gore, Mary was given an unprecedented opportunity at that time to return to the Homer G. nursing school after our baby was born. Also, this course of action happened twice, by Miss. Gore, which allowed Mary to complete nursing school.

Under these circumstances, it makes me wonder if there were some external interventions on Mary's behalf to ensure that she would become a registered nurse. She was destined and determined!

Notes
1. *https://en.wikipedia.org/wiki/Homer_G._Phillips_Hospital*
2. All the information was extracted from *Wikipedia* and is available under the Creative Commons Attribution-Share Alike License.

CHAPTER 11

◇

The Wedding

◇

THERE WAS NO "QUASI-WEDDING PLANNER" to assist with planning our wedding. Mary and I made plans for a small, intimate family wedding. With Mary's approval, most of the wedding arrangements were coordinated by Mrs. Byas, my mother, and me. Each of us agreed to oversee specific arrangements for the wedding.

Mary and I were not stressed out about plans for the wedding. We knew beyond a doubt that we would get married, and that was all that really mattered to us.

We did not mail out wedding invitations. We personally invited a few wedding guests to our private intimate family wedding. Which included our parents, aunts, and close friends, and Mary invited six classmates from Homer G. nursing school.

Almost miraculously, every aspect of our wedding plans was executed daily like clockwork. It was not coincidental or serendipitous that our wedding plans were happening so smoothly. Purchasing Mary's wedding ring-set, getting her wedding gown, obtaining our marriage license, and Reverend Ryce II to perform our marriage ceremony in my home; these events did not occur by happenstance.

Ma Dear To Attend Our Wedding

Less than two weeks before Mary and I were to be married. I came home from work, and in dramatic fashion, mother said, "Momma (Ma Dear) called today, and she is coming to your wedding." Willis, I am so happy that momma will attend your wedding! I know you and Mary will have a blessed wedding and a happy married life together.

I was ecstatic and felt extremely honored. Ma Dear just doesn't travel anymore, and I never expected, at her age and health conditions, that she would attend my wedding. "I feel so blessed, and my emotions stirred inside me."

As a teenager growing up in St. Louis, I did not see my grandmother often. She lived in Memphis, TN, and I would see her in the summertime when we visited her. However, I would write her letters monthly. Ma Dear would respond, now and then, to my letters. Over the years, my mother would tell me "that she had talked to momma, and she said how much joy reading your letters had brought her."

There are numerous "adages" in African-American culture and history. I don't know if this is one of those, but it is true. "Being kind and showing love to someone will result in you receiving love back twofold." I believe as a young teenager, when I wrote letters to Ma Dear monthly, the joy she received over the years inspired her to express her special love for me by attending my wedding."

Talking to Mary that evening, I told her that Ma Dear was coming to our wedding. I often talked to Mary about my grandmother, Ma Dear. Mary was excited, and she understood the significance of Ma Dear's presence at our wedding meant to me. Mary said, "Willis, would you believe our wedding would be this blessed?"

I could sense in her voice the emotions when she said, "Willis, I know we are going to have a beautiful wedding! I can't wait to meet your grandmother." I told Mary that Ma Dear would arrive Wednesday and leave on Saturday. We talked a little longer and finally said good night, and I hit the sack with profound joy in my heart.

The Wedding Ceremony:

Time seemed just to evaporate quickly, and now April 15 was around the corner. On Wednesday afternoon, Ma Dear's brothers, Uncle Jesse and Uncle Big RE, went with me to pick her up from the Union Train Station at 1820 Market Street, St. Louis, MO.

Ma Dear stepped off the train, glancing around, and her brothers greeted their big sister enthusiastically. Uncle Jesse always got emotional seeing his big sister, and tears began to flow from his eyes. Seeing my grandmother was overwhelming, and I just hugged her. We talked as we walked slowly from the train station to the car.

When we got home, mother's emotions spilled over as she embraced her mother. They sat together on the couch in the family room and talked for a little while, and Ma Dear said, "It was a long train ride, and I am going upstairs to rest." Mother told me later that Ma Dear needed to rest because she would prepare and serve the food for my wedding reception dinner.

I immediately called Mary to convey the wonderful news that Ma Dear had arrived this afternoon. Also Ma Dear was going to cater our wedding reception. We didn't talk long, and I whispered good night, "I can't wait two days until Friday to see you." I heard Mary's girlish laughter as we hung up the phone.

I returned downstairs and confirmed with mother if Ma Dear had everything she needed, food-wise, for the reception dinner on Friday. Mother said, "you have bought all of the food, and as we planned, the menu will consist of baked ham, roast beef, potato salad, macaroni and cheese, green beans, I can't remember everything, Willis; yes, homemade rolls and a fruit punch to drink. Don't worry; momma will take care of everything."

I had one day left to work that week as I had scheduled Friday off from work on my wedding day. Thursday at work passed fast, and when I got home from work, I picked up a few food items Ma Dear needed for our wedding reception.

Friday, I woke up at my regular time this morning. Getting out of bed, I stretched and thanked God for another day. With my day off, I wanted to ensure that everything was done that I needed to complete for our wedding ceremony.

I looked out the window, and a smile adorned my face. I realized our wedding day could not have been more perfect weather-wise. There was sunlight, attempting to burst into bright sunshine. The temperature was reasonably warm for the middle of April. My thoughts slowly drifted to what Mary was doing this morning. It was Good Friday, and she had a light class load today.

In keeping with the tradition of do not talk with or see your bride before the wedding ceremony. I was obliged to endure the day in suspense until our wedding ceremony that evening. However, Mary had told me previously that her mother and Aunt Biddy would assist her in getting dressed for her wedding.

There were a few chores mother needed me to do before the wedding. Clean the chandelier in the dining room; take the Chinaware, silverware, and serving utensils from the China cabinet so she can clean them. She wanted to set the dining room table for the reception dinner.

In the morning, I was helping mother, and Ma Dear was in the kitchen preparing food. I finally observed everything in the dining room was done, and I paused and relished in the magnificence of the arrangements that had been done for our wedding reception.

Suddenly I looked at my watch, and panic temporarily surfaced; it was after 2:00 pm. I asked mother if she needed my help any longer. Smiling, "no, Willis, everything is in place the way I want." Let me see if momma needs my help. I walked into the kitchen with mother, and she asked, "Momma can I help you with anything?"

Ma Dear stopped what she was doing, turned, looked at mother, and said, "Wylor Dean, I have prepared for extravagant dinner parties most of my life and for a larger number of guests than this one. No baby, I don't need your help; you would just be in the way.

So you just go sit and rest a while." Mother put her arms around Ma Dear's shoulders, and mother and I both laughed so hard. Mother went and sat down on the couch in her favorite spot, and I retreated upstairs to my bedroom.

I laid down and stretched across the bed, focusing on the fact that in less than four hours, Mary Ann Byas would become my wife, Mrs. Mary Ann Byas-Drake. I started to feel relaxed, and my body was succumbing to the tiredness I now felt. My will was giving in, and I was surrendering to the rest I needed. I submitted to taking at least a short nap.

I heard mother call my name, Willis, Willis, do you know what time it is? I stirred from my nap, answering, yes, mom, I am aware of the time, which I wasn't. I was thankful mother had woken me up. It was now 4:15 pm, and I hurriedly got up.

I had everything organized and proceeded to shower and get dressed more particularly than usual. I looked at myself in the mirror and pro-claimed that I was dressed really sharp, to the nine, and was looking good. It was 5:35 pm, and family members and guests had started to arrive at the house. I was still waiting upstairs so I would not breach the tradition of seeing my bride, Mary, before the wedding ceremony.

My big brother, Charles Edward Drake Sr., came upstairs and told me that Mary had arrived. That her mother and her aunt were in the bed-room putting the finishing touches on Mary's wedding gown.

Charles straightened out my necktie and said I could come downstairs and get ready for the ceremony. Beaming with confidence, I asked Charles how do I look? I wanted my big brother's approval of my appearance. With that broad smile, he said, "Little brother, you look handsome." I responded, "of course, that is understood because all of the Drake men are handsome." He broke out laughing, and I felt relaxed and ready to get married.

We went downstairs, and I passed the front bedroom on the second floor, where Mary was putting the final touches on her wedding gown. Charles and I continued to the first floor, where my best man, Garland Greer, was waiting. We greeted one another and commented on how sharp we both looked. We walked into the living room, waiting for the ceremony to begin.

We were now positioned at our places, and I heard the music "Here comes the bride," Mary descended the staircase and entered the living room. I gasped as I gazed at Mary in her wedding gown that fitted her as if it had been tailor-made specifically for her. She was a beautiful, magnificent-looking bride, and she took her place next to me.

Our wedding ceremony took place at six o'clock in the evening, on April 15, 1960, in the living room at my parents' home, 4462 Enright Avenue, St. Louis, Mo. The living room was not exceptionally large, but it would comfortably accommodate the wedding party, "the Bride, Groom, Best Man, and Reverend Amos Ryce II," plus fifteen guests.

On the left side of the living room, Mary's parents stood close behind her. My mom, dad, grandmother (Ma Dear), and Tee stood close behind me on the right side of the living room. The center of the living room was open to allow the wedding guest to witness the wedding ceremony in the living room and family room areas.

Mary and I were especially blessed to have our parents, favorite aunts (Aunt Mary, Aunt Biddy, and my Aunt Tee), sisters, brothers, best friends, and classmates from the Homer G. nursing school. Besides my grandmother being special, my young nieces and nephews, from ages one to eight, attended our wedding. To this day, it is a day that I have never forgotten.

Reverend Amos Ryce II

The wedding party was facing the living room window, and Reverend Amos Ryce II was facing us. He performed a traditional Christian wedding ceremony, which Mary and I wanted.

He recited words of Scripture from the Holy Bible with the standard Christian Holy Matrimony Vows. The words were similar to the following: "I, Mary Ann Byas, take you, Willis Drake, to be my husband to have and to hold from this day forward, for better for worse, for richer for poorer, in sickness and in health, to love and to cherish, till death do us part, according to God's holy law; and this is my solemn vow."

Mary and I were looking into one another's eyes as Reverend Ryce recited our marriage vows and married us. I still recall the image of how radiant Mary looked standing by my side. To me, Mary was so beautiful waiting to be announced as my wife, Mrs. Mary Ann Byas-Drake, as Reverend Ryce gave us the vows to repeat after him.

The radiance from Mary's smile indicated her true happiness. I cannot attest to what I may have reflected or looked like externally. From my inner being, I know exactly how I felt. Without a doubt, in my mind, I felt complete, with Mary as my wife to be standing by my side.

Now I finally understood my mother's vision, which was revealed to her three years earlier, before I met Mary. My mother's vision was foretold to her when I was only sixteen years old. The Holy Spirit had revealed and confirmed to her three times that this unknown girl at the time, Mary Ann Byas, would be my wife.

As I reflect on our wedding, I knew then and can testify now that we had a blessed and beautiful wedding. I can start with Mary's borrowed wedding dress, which did not require a stitch of alterations, and it fit her perfectly.

After we had recited our vows, Reverend Ryce announced that I could kiss (salute) my bride." I kissed Mary, and the kiss was quite long. Then

Reverend Ryce smiling, told me, "Willis, you have saluted Mary long enough." Everyone, including our parents, laughed. Mary was the most beautiful bride I have ever seen.

There was a personal sentimental moment between Reverend Ryce and me as we shook hands again. He displayed a very firm handshake, and while still grasping my hand, he had a serious look on his face. Then in a fatherly way, he said, "Willis, you take good care of your wife, Mary! She will be a wonderful wife to you." I acknowledged his sentiments and thanked him for everything.

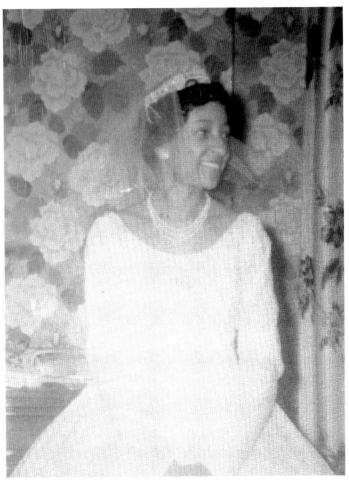

The Wedding Gown: Mary Ann Byas-Drake

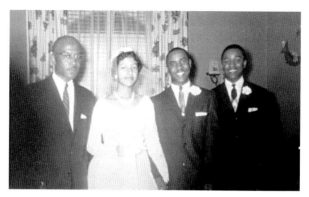

From left to right: Reverend Amos Ryce II, Mary Ann Byas-Drake, Willis Drake, and Garland Greer (Best Man)

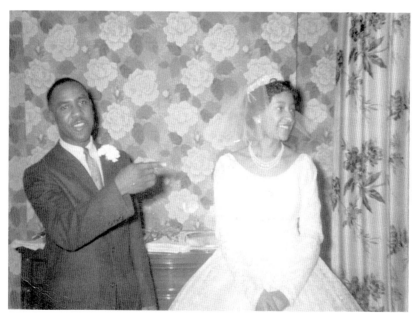

Willis Drake and Mary Ann Byas-Drake.
(In her beautiful wedding dress)

Beforehand, I was completely unaware that Mary would need different attire for the wedding reception. After the wedding ceremony, she would need to change into something casually dressy for the wedding reception. That aspect of our reception, Mary's mother, had that occasion covered too.

The dress Mary wore at the wedding reception was a greenish and bluish multicolor soft fabric material with flower designs. It had puffed sleeves that fit at her shoulders and a low square shape neckline aligned with the puffed sleeves. The waistline of the dress fitted tightly on her waist. From the waist down, the dress flared out, fitting her loosely. Mary looked beautiful in that dress as well.

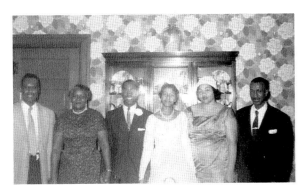

The photo from left to right: Kermit Drake Sr., Wylor Dean Drake, Willis Drake, Mary Ann Byas-Drake, Ruby Byas, and Matthew Byas

Tossing the Flower Bouquet:
Mary had every aspect of a "traditional wedding ceremony" as part of our wedding ceremony. She had the traditional flower bouquet toss standing on the stairwell platform, with her back turned to the eligible young ladies, all of her classmates. Mary tossed her flower bouquet over her left shoulder.

Mary's Homer G. classmate, Floydie Addison's emotional expression after catching the flower bouquet added to the excitement of our memorable wedding.

Twenty-five years later, when Mary and I moved to Virginia, we reconnected with Floydie and Ed Scott, her husband. We joined the St. Louis Club of Washington DC, which they were members of. Mary gave Floydie a copy of the picture of her catching Mary's flower bouquet at our wedding.

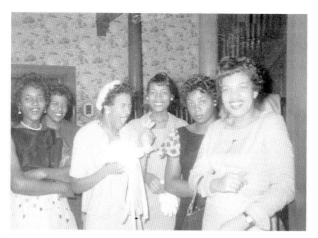

The photo from left to right: Dorothy Wilson, Marva Shegog, Floydie Addison-Scott, (Unknown name), Florence Jean Charleston-Washington and Constance (Connie) Fitzpatrick.

The Wedding Reception

Initially, I didn't have a clue that Ma Dear was going to cater our wedding reception. Her presence at our wedding was a great honor and blessing for me.

Ma Dear seldom traveled from Memphis anymore. She was seventy-two years old now, and her mobility was somewhat impaired. She had not traveled any distance from Memphis since she came to St. Louis seven years ago for her younger brother; Jesse (Johnson) Smith's wedding in 1953. It was astonishing to me that Ma Dear would travel on a train alone, from Memphis to St. Louis, at this stage of her life to attend our wedding.

Mary and I were not financially situated to have an exorbitant or even a very modest wedding reception. However, I assured Mary that we would have a blessed, enjoyable, and wonderful reception. Mother had arranged for the wedding reception dinner to start immediately following the wedding ceremony.

We followed the tradition of many African-American weddings. After Mary had tossed her flower bouquet, we then celebrated in the feast my grandmother had prepared for our wedding reception dinner.

It was phenomenal that Mary and I were fortunate enough to have Ma Dear, an experienced "caterer," to cater our wedding reception. She planned every detail to ensure that our wedding reception would be first-class, in fact, exceptional. Her overall experience and expertise included food preparation, decorating, and arranging the table setting, and how to serve food in a professional and special way.

Ma Dear had worked most of her life as a domestic housekeeper for a well-known real estate manager, Harry Dermon (the Dermon Building in downtown Memphis, Tennessee, is named after the family). She was recognized for preparing some of the most elegant and elite dinner parties and social affairs in Memphis while working for the Dermons.

Ma Dear's wedding gift to Mary and I was attending our wedding and "catering" our wedding reception. Her presence also added elegance to the reception and provided a spiritual reflection that I will always remember. My parent's home had a large formal dining room, which would accommodate a twelve-person dinner setting.

Mother also had the Chinaware and Silverware necessary to host an elegant, if not an elaborate, dinner party or wedding reception. Our reception was not a buffet or serve-yourself affair. We were blessed with a full-course meal consisting of five courses. It was a first-class sit-down reception dinner. Ma Dear personally served each dinner course of the meal to the dinner guest.

Every time I see the picture of Ma Dear serving the dinner guest during our wedding reception, it ignites the gratitude, appreciation, and love that I felt for my grandmother and her for me. Ma Dear's presence at our wedding and her wedding reception gift was an expression of her love for Mary and me.

To conclude the reception dinner party, Mary and I cut our wedding cake in traditional fashion, and then we got ready for "party" time.

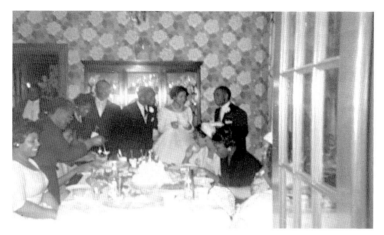

The photo from left to right: Mildred (Aunt Biddy) Thomas,
Ma Dear (L. A. Sanford), Charles Drake Sr., Dorothy Wilson,
Shirley Drake-Sykes, Cleart Jones, Garland Greer, Mary Ann Byas-Drake,
Willis Drake, Floydie Addison, Marva Shegog,
Ruby Byas (Mary's mother), Mary Tolden (Aunt Mary).

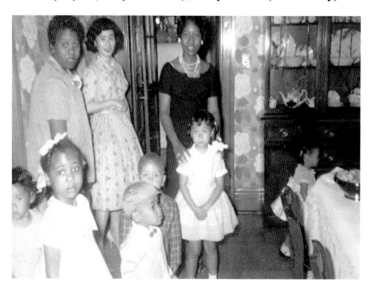

The photo from left to right: Front row—Paula Drake,
Musette Burnham, Wayne Gooch, Flarzell Harris Jr., Shirley Drake
(Little Shirley), Arcola (Queenie) Drake, Back row: Joan Drake-Harris,
Mihoko Drake, Shirley Drake-Sykes.

Following an exquisite reception dinner, our parents, and adult relatives (Ma Dear (L A Sanford), Aunt Mary (Mary Tolden), Aunt Biddy (Mildred Thomas), and Ethel Mae Sanford (Tee)) retired for the evening.

My young nieces and nephews (Charles Drake Jr., (Little) Shirley Drake, Paula Drake, Arcola (Queenie) Drake, Musette Burnham, Ricky Gill, Wayne Gooch, and Flarzell Harris) after they had witnessed Mary and my marriage ceremony and participated in the wedding reception for a brief time (eating cake and ice cream) they too departed.

Reception Party Time:
Mary changed out of her wedding gown into her reception dress. Now we were ready to celebrate with Mary's classmates, members of the Tandy boxing team, family members, and friends.

As beautiful as Mary looked in her wedding gown and reception dress, her heart was even happier internally. Mary and I had our first dance, and then there was a celebration toast "wishing us a happy marriage."

Now the reception had shifted into full swing, and it was celebration time. The reception became much larger than we had planned. Friends from the old neighborhood came to the house and congratulated Mary and me on our marriage.

We had the latest popular music records to play on my Hi-Fi, and we danced and had a great time. We had hors d'oeuvre, snacks, finger food to eat, drink refreshments, and desserts. We celebrated big time, and Mary's classmates enjoyed the wedding ceremony and reception. They were also able to party until 10:30 pm when they had to leave to meet their 11:00 pm weekend curfew. At that time, when our guests were leaving, Mary and I retired to the boudoir!

Mary and I did not have a formal honeymoon. First, we could not afford it, and also Mary had to be back at the nursing dormitory by her curfew time Sunday at 11:00 pm. Mary and I enjoyed Saturday and Sunday as our honeymoon time.

After the Wedding

Unfortunately, Mrs. Byas' friend, that loaned Mary her wedding gown could not attend our wedding. On Easter Sunday afternoon, two days after our wedding, we returned the wedding dress to Mary's mother's friend.

It was a beautiful day that Easter Sunday afternoon as Mary and I left my house and walked across Taylor Avenue holding hands. This was the same Taylor Avenue that Mary and I had walked on that frigid cold evening that created "The Walk" and, in my mind, confirmed the love Mary and I shared for each other.

Unlike that December evening, the weather was great this Easter Sunday afternoon. Mary and I crossed Finney Avenue, where I used to live. Walking fast, we were only five minutes away from arriving at Evans Avenue.

Mary's mother's friend lived in the 4400 block of Evans Avenue, seven blocks north of my house. It was only ten or fifteen minutes' walking distance from where I lived. She stayed in a house on the north side of Evans Avenue, the second or third house East of Taylor Avenue.

Now standing on the front porch, I rang the doorbell, and almost immediately, a lady opened the door. She and Mary were about the same height. She had a medium dark-brown skin complexion and had a pleasant smile.

She invited us to step inside the house, and she gave Mary a tight hug. Mary introduced me, saying, "This is my husband, Willis Drake." We greeted one another, and Mary and I sincerely thanked her for using the beautiful wedding gown. With a big smile, she told Mary, "I have known Ruby, your mother since we were youngsters. I am so pleased that you were able to wear the wedding gown.

Also, my husband and I have had a blessed marriage for many years now, and I pray you and Willis will also." She then looked at me and said, "Ruby told me you are a very fine young man." She hugged me and again offered her best wishes for a blessed and happy marriage to Mary and me. Unfortunately, I couldn't recall her name at this point, as that was over fifty-five wonderful years ago.

Living With My Aunt, Tee

When we got married, we were living at my parent's home, and we lived there for the first two weeks after we were married. My Aunt Tee lived alone, and my mother, Tee's sister, was concerned for her safety living by herself. Mother suggested, "That Mary and I should consider living with your Aunt Tee, and I know she would be delighted to have you live with her."

Mary and I discussed the situation, and Mary said, "She would be comfortable living with Tee in her apartment." Mary and I met with Tee and discussed "if we could rent the vacant bedroom in her apartment and live with her while Mary was in nursing school. Tee was very fond of Mary and me.

Tee enthusiastically said, "yes, Willis! You and Mary are welcome to live here with me." Mary was sitting on the couch next to Tee, and they hugged. I told Tee that we should discuss all the agreements and conditions for us to live with you. That way, we will understand the living agreement and arrangements from the start.

Tee laughed and said, "Willis, you were always looking ahead to ensure things were laid out properly. We agreed on the modest rent that included the utilities and that we would pay our rent monthly. We would have use of the total apartment, which included the kitchen and the living room. Mary and I would purchase and cook our own food.

When we left Tee's house that day, Mary and I completely understood the arrangements for us to live with Tee comfortably. We agreed to move into the apartment on May 1, 1960.

CHAPTER 12

—— ◇ ——

Married—Attending Nursing School

—— ◇ ——

Tee's apartment was completely furnished, except for a television in the back bedroom. Tee occupied the front master bedroom, and Mary and I would occupy the back bedroom. This was also the same bedroom I slept in when I was a young kid living in this house (apartment).

The living room was fashionably decorated with modern contemporary-style furniture, and the kitchen was modestly furnished. Mary and I had access to the living room and the kitchen. I started bringing our clothes and personal items to Tee's apartment early during the week.

We had space for our clothes in the dresser drawers and the hall closet for our hang-up clothes. It didn't take us long that weekend to get organized and settled into the apartment. When Mary came home from school Friday evening, she came to Tee's apartment, our new home.

Mary and I had everything we needed in the apartment except a Television (TV). The next weekend, Mary and I went downtown to Famous and Barr Department store on Saturday and purchased a TV. When the TV was delivered, our apartment was now complete.

Basically, Mary's weekend routine did not change. The difference was that she would come home to our apartment instead of going to her parent's home on the weekend. However, she still had to adhere to the dormitory curfew. Our time together was so precious. It seemed that 11:00 pm Sunday rolled around so quickly. I would wait until the very last minute to take Mary back to the dormitory.

Mary being a newlywed, a student, and an expecting mother was a tremendous emotional challenge for her. Adjusting to handle her emotional adjustments and staying focused on school was an extremely exigent situation for her. As newlyweds, it was necessary that Mary and I stay focused; she maintained passing grades in her classes.

The fact that Mary only came home on the weekends complicated the situation somewhat. She would tell me, "Willis, I cannot stop counting the days, Monday through Friday, and anticipating coming home for the weekend. I know I have to stay focused more on my classes to maintain passing grades, but it's not easy."

I tried to keep Mary uplifted, so I concealed from her that, similarly, not seeing her during the week was also very tough for me. During the week, I would anticipate when the weekend would come so we could be together.

The natural effort was immense for Mary as we balanced our emotions, and she focused on finishing the school semester on an elevated level. When we got married, it was understood that she would definitely continue nursing school. It was both a personal and spiritual obligation for her. When Mrs. Byas and I discussed before my marriage to Mary, I gave her my "word" that I would do everything possible for Mary to complete nursing school.

After two weeks of this routine, Mary and I decided that she would come home on Wednesday evenings, so we could spend time together. That way, we would have only two consecutive days of not seeing one another; instead of being apart for five straight days. This new arrangement reduced our individual stress tremendously.

Mary's Financial Aid From the State of Illinois

It was the end of May, and Mary came home for the weekend. She was direct, "Willis, we need to discuss the financial obligation I have with the State of Illinois. I am not sure what prompted her to raise this discussion or if it was sort of initiated by happenstance. Regardless it was a conversation we needed to have.

Mary explained that "When I started nursing school, I got a financial aid grant from the state of Illinois to finance my nursing education. The state grant paid my tuition costs, and I receive a fifteen dollars weekly stipend that provides funds for my incidental expenses.

The condition for my grant specified that after graduating from nursing school, I would be obligated to work as a registered nurse in the state of Illinois for a state or city agency for three years. Willis, I had received approximately fifteen hundred dollars ($1,500.) in payments from the grant.

I know we will be living in St. Louis, and hopefully, I will get a nurse's position working in the City." The next week we terminated her grant agreement, and we started repaying the state of Illinois the funds Mary had received. By the next year, we had repaid the loan, and Mary was released from all obligations she had to the Illinois State government for employment purposes.

Signs of Morning Sickness

Mary was having "Morning Sickness" symptoms. One evening she called me, and she was extremely upset. "Willis, this morning, I was notified by the student nurse's administration office that I was scheduled to get a physical examination today. I went for the physical, and the doctor used his stethoscope to listen to my stomach; he apparently was trying to determine if I was pregnant. He commented, "you have gained weight since your last physical. Are you feeling okay?"

Mary was disturbed. "She was very annoyed with that stupid old doctor, and I told him I felt fine." I was ticked off from having the examination, and I immediately went and talked with Miss Gore, the Nursing Director.

I told her, "If the doctor had just asked me, I would have told him that I was pregnant," she reiterated. Miss Gore apologized on behalf of the doctor and said, "I will talk with the medical staff, so you will not have any more physical examinations." As Mary finished telling me of the situation, she was calm, and we had a normal time that evening.

Mary's Determination
Mary was locked in and determined to keep superb grades in all her classes. Coming home on Wednesdays and even on the weekends, it sometimes was difficult for her to stay focused on studying. We would "accidentally on purpose" distract one another when we were together.

It was obvious that we immensely enjoyed being at home together. We would have fun laughing and just being together as newlyweds. It was out of sight. When Mary had to concentrate totally and study for a serious exam, she would not come home on Wednesday during the week.

Not surprisingly, working towards completing her first year of nursing school, Mary fulfilled her freshman goals with excellent grades. Week by week, her weekend routine had become more normalized. Her academic confidence also increased as she was among the class academic leaders.

It seemed that July had appeared instantly, and the school year was nearing its end. Mary was obviously perplexed about how to proceed with the Director of Nursing, Miss. Gore, regarding if she would allow her to return to HGP for her junior year of nursing school.

Mary's Discussion With Miss. Gore
Now it was Monday morning, the 4th of July. Mary said, "Willis, tomorrow I am going to talk with Miss. Gore, so I can find out after our baby is born if she will allow me to return to Homer G. for my junior year of school in August 1961.

Instantaneously Mary stated, "We are invited to celebrate the 4th of July with your parents. I plan to eat plenty of barbecue ribs, sides of potato salad, Mac & Cheese, baked beans, coleslaw, and cake." On most holidays during the day, mother's children living in the city would stop by her house.

Family members started filing in the house around 2:30 pm that day. We ate barbecue, shot off fireworks, and enjoyed the holiday celebration with our family. We said our goodbyes to the family around 8:00 pm. Mary had to return to the Homer G. dormitory by 11:00 pm tonight.

As we were driving to the dorm, Mary said, "Baby, wish me luck when I talk with Miss. Gore." I squeezed her left hand affectively as our signal to say you know I am with you 100%! Now at the dormitory, I watched Mary enter the building, and I drove away and was back home in twenty minutes.

With Monday being a holiday, we had a short four-day workweek. However, our routine was the same, our nightly phone calls and the anticipation of Mary coming home Friday evening. This Friday seemingly had arrived so quickly.

When Mary walked into the house that evening, she was exuberant. She greeted me very amorously. With her arms around my neck, she kissed me passionately. I did not know the reason for her excitement, but I returned her kiss with the same passionate intensity.

At the end of the school year, Mary had her requested "exit review" consultation with Miss. Gore. Mary did not know if this was standard protocol or not for a nursing student to have an exit interview with the Director of Nursing.

However, Mary had a unique circumstance of being married and expecting a baby in four months. To contemplate her future at the HGP Nursing School, Mary's unique situation required deliberation with Miss. Minnie Edythe Todd Gore. Who would decide if Mary could return to HGP nursing school for her junior year of school.

Mary said she and Miss. Gore had a very candid discussion about her first year of nursing school. Then Miss. Gore asked me, "what my plans were after my baby is born?"

"Willis, I was surprised at Miss. Gore's question and her candor. Then I shared my hopes and expectations with her, and tears welled in my eyes. I let her know that I want to be a nurse. That after our baby is born, "I very much want to return to Homer G. and finish HGP nursing school and become a registered nurse," Mary continued.

Mary was a little emotional at this point, and she sat down in the chair. "Willis, Miss Gore's very straightforward, candid conversation with me was straight-up. She told me just how difficult she thought it would be for me to finish nursing school with a young baby.

Willis, I was getting concerned regarding the detailed questions Miss. Gore were posing to me. Then a peaceful calm came over me. I explained that my mother would keep my baby during the week. My husband and I will take care of our baby on the weekends. He will care for our baby when I am studying on weekends."

Mary was now smiling and said, "Willis, I agreed with Miss. Gore that it will not be easy being a mother and a full-time student nurse. However, I told her, "if you allow me to return to school for my junior school year, I know I will be successful."

"Willis, Miss. Gore looked at me sternly as we were talking. She said, 'Mrs. Drake, I have seriously considered your situation.' Looking me directly in my eyes, she said, 'before having this conversation with you, I had decided to hold your nurse's position open for you to return to the HGP nursing program after your baby was born.'"

Note 1: Miss. Gore was appointed in 1951 as the director of nursing at HGP. She had a bachelor's degree in nursing education, plus a Master's degree and some work towards a doctorate. She proved to be a powerful force in the hospital's history. While some students found her daunting or even unfriendly, others described her as strict but fair and often very kind. Unquestionably, Mary's feelings fell into the latter category.

"Willis, hearing Miss Gore tell me that I can return to nursing school after our baby is born was overwhelming. I fought back the tears, but my eyes watered up, and I cried unashamedly. I thanked Miss. Gore and I told her, "I greatly appreciated her giving me this opportunity, and I am so grateful.""

Miss. Gore said I am an excellent student and have human compassion to be a wonderful nurse. She acknowledged that she was taking a chance on me, but she knew I would not let her down. she said she had not made this type of student exception before."

I am not certain if Mary was aware then that her mother had an in-depth conversation with Miss. Gore on Mary's behalf, regarding her returning to Homer G. after our baby was born. If she knew, she never mentioned it to me.

Mrs. Ruby Byas and Miss. Minnie Edith T. Gore Talk

Mary completed her first year of nursing school in July 1960 and was now resolved to be a housewife and mother-to-be. Our baby was due in late November 1960. Under normal circumstances, Mary would not have been granted the opportunity to retain her "student nursing position" and return to Homer G. nursing school to continue her education a year later.

Homer G. was a fully accredited student nursing training program. Its reputation throughout the country was far-reaching among African-Americans wanting to become registered nurses.

We visited Mary's parents shortly after she finished her first year of nursing school. Mary's mother and I casually conversed in the living room. In her serious but humorous way, she told me, "before Pookie finished her freshman year of nursing school; I had a meeting with Miss. Gore, the Homer G. Phillips Director of Nursing, to ask her to allow "Pookie" to return to school after her baby is born.

She said, "Willis, I honestly pleaded with Miss. Gore to permit Pookie to return to nursing school after her baby is born. Miss. Gore and I talked for over an hour, and I poured my heart out to her.

I explained to Miss. Gore how Pookie (Mary) has always wanted to be a nurse. I practically begged her to allow Pookie (Mary) a chance to return to school and finish the Homer G. nursing program.

Willis, Miss. Gore listened to me intently and politely but stoically. Then she spoke passionately and acknowledged that Mary (Pookie) was an excellent student nurse. Now hearing Mary's story, she appreciates Mary's deep love for the nursing profession. She now understands how Mary would get so emotionally attached to her patients, which was hard for her to overcome at one point."

I digested every word Mrs. Byas shared with me. I marveled at the thought of how she pleaded her daughter Pookie's case, telling Mary's story to Miss. Gore. I don't know what exact words were spoken between Mrs. Byas and Miss. Gore during what had to be a phenomenal honest and passionate conversation. I can only speculate that it was a heartfelt discussion.

Also, I do not know about Miss. Gore's spiritual beliefs. However, I can imagine that in the midst of Mrs. Byas and Miss. Gore's conversation, there was a spiritual component advocating on Mary's behalf and one that touched Miss. Gore's heart.

When situations happen that I do not understand, I subscribe to and accept the fact. In this case, specifically, the presence of the Holy Spirit ensured that Mary's desire to become a nurse would be fulfilled.

Miss. Gore, on that day, committed to Mrs. Byas that she would keep Mary's student nursing position available until Mary completed the Homer G. nursing program. It is important to understand the significance of the commitment that Miss. Gore made to Mary.

Her decision was bolstered because Mary was an outstanding student with excellent grades. The assumption is that Mary's grades were a factor, and it provided Miss. Gore the support she needed to secure Mary's nursing position in a future class.

Note 2: Miss. Gore, in 1960, allowed Mary Ann Byas-Drake to be married and return to HGP nursing school. This predates the decision that "A handful (students) got special dispensation to marry during training." Our class was the first that they allowed a student to get married," said a student in the class of 1966."

Listening to Mrs. Byas revealing the salient details of that conversation between her and Miss. Gore, concerning Mary's nursing future, was compelling. I believe the right people were put in Mary's life at the right time to fulfill her dream of becoming a registered nurse. She was destined and determined.

Tee, Mary, and I
Our living arrangements with Tee were very convenient for the three of us. Tee didn't have children; however, she had always been part of our family. She was a "true" aunt to her nieces and nephews.

Mary and I had been living with Tee for three months, and Mary had just completed her freshman year of nursing school. It was the end of July, and Mary was now home all week and adjusting to being a housewife. Tee and Mary had formed a close aunt and niece bond between them.

Now being a non-student, one of Mary's first undertakings was to prepare a "family" meal. It was Tee's off day, and when I got home from work, Mary greeted me as usual with a smile and a kiss.

She said, "Willis, I hope you are hungry; I fixed your favorite meal for dinner." Grinning profusely, I walked into the kitchen. "Whatever you are cooking smells really good," I replied. "I hope you like it, babe. Hurry and wash up so we can eat before the food gets cold," she continued. I quickly washed my face and hands and returned to the kitchen, ready to eat.

Tee, Mary, and I sat down at the dinner table, and I blessed the food. Mary had cooked spaghetti, fried fish, coleslaw, deviled eggs, and garlic bread, and, of course, orange juice to drink. We ate dinner together as a family, just laughing and talking. I ate more than usual, and I praised Mary for a wonderful dinner when we finished eating. This was the best meal she had ever cooked for me. Mary appreciated my sincere compliments, and it showed on her smiling face.

I sat at the table as Tee and Mary cleaned the kitchen and put the leftover food in the refrigerator. Tee hugged Mary and said, "Willis, I am so happy you and Mary are living with me. We have our little family, and I enjoy my days off when we have dinner together. Mary, you know I don't spend much time in the kitchen, and I appreciate you cooking dinner this evening."

Mary, laughing, told Tee, "don't praise me too soon about my cooking. I am still learning, but I do enjoy cooking. Tee, I appreciate how you have made me feel so welcome living here with you." I echoed Mary's sentiments, "Tee, you have accepted Mary as one of your nieces, and I appreciate that." "Willis, I love Mary the same as I love all my nieces," Tee responded.

With the kitchen cleaned up, I went to watch TV. Tee and Mary sat at the kitchen table, talking about Mary returning to school for her junior year after the baby is born. I could hear their laughter as I watched the evening news. After the news was off, Tee went to her room, and Mary and I watched TV until bedtime.

$\diamond$

Birth of Willis Jr.

$\diamond$

T HE MENTAL BURDEN WAS NOW removed from her mind, knowing she would be returning to school in August 1961 for her junior year. Mary was eager to enjoy married life and anticipated having our baby in November. That first weekend after she had completed school, Mary decided we should get outside and enjoy the beautiful July weather.

That Sunday afternoon, Mary persuaded my sister, Jean, to go with us to Forest Park and get out in the fresh air. We rode the bus to Forest Park. Mary was five months pregnant, and she looked so beautiful. Her countenance was radiant, so vibrant, and she had a glow about her that was breathtaking.

She wore khaki color Bermuda shorts and a brown multicolored short-sleeve blouse. Mary and I were holding hands, enjoying a beautiful day walking in the park. Jean and Mary were acting like sisters. It reminded me of when Jean, Joan, Shirley, and I were kids, and mother would take us to Forest Park.

Now it felt great taking a carefree stroll in the park with Mary. When I looked at her, knowing we were going to have a baby in four months; generated astonishing thoughts within me. That outing was the most exhilarating since Mary and I walked together on Easter Sunday after our wedding. We walked through the zoo and picnic area, and as the evening drew near, we caught the bus and returned home.

During the ensuing weeks and month-to-month during her pregnancy, Mary was healthy as her delivery time got closer. She had the usual morning sickness symptoms early on. She didn't have any dire food cravings that required me to go out at odd night hours to satisfy her cravings.

Mary's delivery date was close, and we had gone to bed Saturday night at 9:30. At 2:30 am Sunday, Mary woke me up and said, "Willis, I am ready to go to the hospital. The baby is ready to come."

Fortunately, Tee was off work and helped Mary get dressed. The Allen Taxicab I ordered arrived to take us to Firmin Desloge Hospital on Grand between Vista Avenue and Rutgers Avenues. There was little traffic that early in the morning driving to the hospital. The cab driver asked how she was doing.

He apparently understood the gravity and urgency of the situation. We arrived at the emergency hospital entrance within fifteen minutes; an emergency hospital attendant rushed to help Mary from the taxicab and into a wheelchair.

I was walking alongside, holding her hand. The hospital admission nurse summoned the doctor. Mary let him know her labor pains were 10 to 15 minutes apart. Mary was immediately taken to the examination room.

Thirty minutes later, the doctor informed me, "Your wife is resting comfortably. However, it likely would be hours before she will have the baby. She is in a sterile area, so you cannot see her now. I will update you frequently on her status."

It was now six o'clock in the morning, and I called Mrs. Byas and told her, "Mary was in the hospital, but the doctor thinks it will be several hours before the baby is born." Mrs. Byas entered the waiting room at seven o'clock and sat next to me. I told her that Mary was in labor, but she was experiencing some difficulty.

Mary was in labor for a considerable time before our son was born. Thanks to the doctors, and we know through the grace of God, our son was born a healthy baby, and Mary came through childbirth in good health too. Our son was born on Sunday, November 27, 1960, at 10:40 am. He weighed 7 lbs, 7 ounces and his length was 23 inches, and we named him Willis Jr., and he was a blessing to our family.

Day by day, Mary was slowly regaining her strength, and I was able to bring her and Willis Jr. home on Thursday afternoon. When we came into the house, Tee said, "Willis let me take the baby, and you help Mary." We went to our bedroom, and Mary sat in the chair. She said, "Tee, I will take the baby now."

Tee looking at Willis Jr., said, "He looks so intelligent, and I can tell he is going to be a smart child." Tee carefully handed Mary her baby. Mary started "cooing" and making baby talk "soft murmuring sounds," with Willis Jr. nesting in her arms as she rocked him back and forth. Continuing to talk to him as if he understood every word she was saying.

I was observing my young wife's motherly instincts kicking in, knowing how to care for her baby. Possibly it was her nurse training, but logically, it was an innate maternal gift that all mothers inherently possess. Instantly, Mary looked happy sitting in the chair, cradling her baby in her arms.

When Mary was in the hospital, Tee cleaned and sterilized the bedroom and the kitchen, and they were spotlessly clean. Mary said, "Baby, the hospital gave me two eight-ounce bottles of milk formula to bring home to feed the baby. Did you put it in the refrigerator?" "Yes, I did, and if he gets hungry, we will have milk to feed him," I responded.

Mary had been sitting in the chair for thirty minutes now. She called Tee to come and hold Willis Jr. so she could get up and put him in his baby crib. Tee was immediately at Mary's side, and she took the baby from Mary's arms and carefully laid him in his baby crib.

Mary said, "I am tired, and I want to lay down and rest too. She then commented, telling Tee, "that baby crib has been passed down through the family, as the siblings had babies. That's the baby crib that Maudean initially bought for her baby Musette (Burnham), and then Wayne Gooch, Richard Gill (Musette's brother), and now Willis Jr. is using the baby crib."

Tee said, "Mary, Maud (Maudean) always purchased high-quality items, and that baby crib still looks great. I know you will take care of it also, for the next baby in the family to use. They laughed, and Mary echoed, "Tee, I will definitely take care of the baby crib like the family heirloom it is."

Tee left the room, and Mary quickly put on her nightgown, and I helped her get comfortable into bed. I kissed her and told her to get some rest. Okay, I am going to sleep now while the baby is sleeping. I told Mary I would keep my eye on the baby while she slept. That was the first day in our apartment that Mary and I were parents responsible for our son, Willis Jr.'s well-being.

Mary had given me the list of supplies we needed to make the baby's milk formula, and I had written out the process and put it in the kitchen work area. I went into the kitchen and started making the baby's milk formula. It will take an hour for the baby's milk to be ready.

I had purchased a milk formula maker, which would make six eight-ounce bottles of milk formula at once. Mary said, "To use canned "Pet Evaporated Milk" with the proper water ratio and add a pinch of Karo Syrup for sweetness. Then the formula was boiled for 45 minutes in the six individual baby milk bottles, and now we would have the milk to feed Willis Jr. on a planned schedule.

Our Families'—New Baby
I had five days of being home to help take care of our son. Mary was recovering slowly, but she was regaining her strength. That first day

home, she was in bed resting as I watched over our son like a proud father. I stood at his baby crib, admiring him as he was sleeping.

I also observed Mary sleeping, and I thought about the strenuous childbirth she had delivering our son. I could tell that she was still physically uncomfortable. Therefore, I hoped she would sleep until she was well-rested.

Mary woke up several hours later. I said, "Hi, babe; how do you feel now?" With a half-forced smile on her face, "I feel slightly rested, but I am still somewhat uncomfortable. What time is it? Willis, I have to be careful not to move too fast getting in and out of bed.

Did the baby wake up while I was sleeping?" A worried look crossed her face as she became concerned if Willis Jr. had slept okay and had been fed while she was asleep. I was smiling as I assured her that the baby was still asleep and it was not his feeding time yet.

"He should wake up shortly, babe, and I know he will be hungry and ready to eat. Mary was smiling more naturally now. Okay, I will get up, so I can feed and hold my baby when he wakes up," she concluded.

My being home for five days was crucial for Mary to get rest and regain her strength. By Sunday, before I had to return to work on Monday, Mary was able to get up during the early morning to feed and change Willis Jr. She could also now get in and out of bed without my help. Her independence gave me confidence that I could return to work Monday morning without being concerned.

Mary was sufficiently able to take care of the baby, and Tee was also home during the day if Mary needed her help. Willis Jr. was now the "kingpin" in the house. Our new daily routine was built around his sleep, feeding time, and the time he was awake and wanted to be held.

Willis Jr. was one-and-a-half weeks old, and Mary's parents had not seen him since he came home from the hospital. However, they were euphoric about their first grandchild. Mary's mom and dad were coming to see their grandson on Sunday. The jubilance of the birth of their grandson was fully understandable.

My parents and family were also excited about Willis Jr. being born because he was my first child. However, he was their fourteenth grandchild, and they had experienced the joy of being first-time grandparents of their grandchildren many times over.

Mary's parents and her fourteen-year-old cousin, Corliss Byas, came Sunday afternoon to see Willis Jr. I still remember the proud look on Mr. Byas' face as he held his grandson in his arms. I can only imagine the blessing he said over his grandson as he embraced him in his arms. It was also special to Mary that her cousin Corliss came to see our baby.

They had been visiting for several hours, and it was getting late; Mrs. Byas said, "Matt Byas, we had better head back across the bridge." Mary's spirits were lifted tremendously from seeing her mom and dad holding and cuddling their grandson. We said our goodbyes as they were leaving, and Mary was holding Willis Jr. and smiling down at him.

Pictures of Willis Jr. on the Job

I was the epitome of a new dad. At work, I gave my close friends a cigar and acted like any new proud father would, showing them pictures of my son. I also showed Willis Jr.'s picture to Mr. Hamilton and the people in the personnel office.

Willis Jr. was getting bigger as time rolled into December and approaching January. Mary was regaining her strength and was fast returning to her old vibrant self. She had quickly adjusted to being a young mother and homemaker and relished taking care of her baby.

Mary was a typical young mother, and we were learning on the fly. We had plenty of help from our experienced parents in caring for our baby. We had innate parenting instincts and plain common sense. Mostly that is how we managed to take care of our new baby.

However, we would run to the hospital emergency room if Willis Jr. had a slightly elevated temperature. As Mary settled into her motherly role, we both started to react like "normal" young parents. We were not as excitable about the least unusual things like an elevated temperature that we could take care of ourselves.

Mary had assimilated into her motherly role so adequately. It was so natural for her to be a mom. We were homebound most of the time as the winter months slowly passed. Mary utilized her time mostly in teaching Willis Jr. something new every day.

Mary Nicknames Willis Jr., Birdie
During this time, Mary gave Willis Jr. his nickname "Birdie." "When she fed him his milk, he would open his mouth like a baby bird to take his bottle. Therefore, Mary started calling him "Birdie." Still today, his family and friends call him Birdie. I always called my son "Willis."

As the spring of the year approached, Mary psychologically was starting to prepare herself primarily from being around Birdie day in and day out. Mary would periodically say, "Willis, it's getting close to when I will return to nursing school. Her maternal instincts were very keen, and she started to express how she would miss her baby, "Birdie."

Mary was now starting to process the total ramifications of what was required for her to return to Homer G. Nursing School in the coming semester. However, she wanted to make the transition easy for Birdie, being away from her during the entire week. That separation would be a tremendous adjustment for both her and him.

April was now upon us, and the weather was getting warmer. In the evenings, Mary would intermittently digress from her regular daily activities. She would review her nursing materials frequently to keep alert of her nursing knowledge.

Often on the weekends, we would go to Mary's parent's home to visit. We wanted Birdie to become familiar with his grandparents, uncles, and aunts. During the weekdays, when Mary returned to school, her mother would be keeping Birdie the entire week.

This weekend was an enjoyable visit, as always. It was getting late, and we needed to get home before Birdie became irritable. Mary said, "I will have to bathe, feed, and put Birdie to bed as soon as we get home. He has enjoyed himself playing, and he is worn out." Mary hugged and kissed her sisters and brothers as we were leaving the house.

On the way home, surprisingly, Mary said, "Willis, I plan to get a job working in a hospital before I return to nursing school in August. I talked with Tee, and she agreed that it would be prudent for me to get back into the hospital mindset before I started the school semester.

It was obvious that Mary had already obtained Tee's support on this topic. I simply said, "baby; I don't want to get distracted while I am driving. Let's talk about this when we get home, okay?"

Arriving home, Birdie was tuckered out, and Mary bathed and put him to bed. We retreated to our quiet space, the kitchen, and Mary explained her logic for wanting to work in a hospital before returning to nursing school.

Working at Barnes Hospital
Mary was direct to the point. "Willis, to prepare for returning to nursing school, I have been reading my nursing books, literature, and old test papers. Now I think it will be beneficial for me to work in a hospital environment for a month or two before I return to school."

I don't want to be so rusty starting my junior year, having been out of nursing school for a year. Being away from clinical involvement in hospital situations can be an impairment for a junior, second-year nursing student.

Therefore I plan to work the evening shift, so we will not have a major babysitting concern. We will only need a babysitter to keep Birdie from when I go to work until you get home from work. It will only be for a few hours each day.

However, after you get home from work, you will have to feed, bathe, play with, and put Birdie to bed. I laughed, "Baby, that is exactly what I do every night now. That's not a problem if you want to work," I responded.

I will ask Mother Drake if she will babysit Birdie for us. I think Tee may have already mentioned it to her. Mary talked with mother, and she agreed to babysit Birdie when she gets a job. Mary applied for a job at Barnes Hospital and was interviewed on the spot and hired immediately. Mary said the nursing supervisor that interviewed her was impressed with her training as a student nurse at HGP nursing school.

Mary was hired and started as an assistant nurse rather than a Nurse's Aide position. Mary requested to work the evening shift from 3:00 pm to 11:30 pm, and everything was falling into place like a perfect plan.

Birdie was six months old, and Mary had him on a repetitive schedule conducive to her student nurse's schedule routine when she returned to school in August. Mary walking with Birdie in his stroller; it would take her 10 minutes to walk the four blocks to mother's house.

Mary would catch the Taylor bus at Delmar and Taylor avenues, five minutes from mother's house, and in 20 minutes, she would arrive at Barnes Hospital for work on Euclid Avenue. Mother would babysit Birdie from 2:00 pm until 4:30 pm each evening.

On the job, Mary was quickly back in her nursing element. Day by day, the hospital environment seemed to stimulate and put her into the academic mode of learning. She was enjoying being in nursing situations again, and it was obvious that her job motivated her to get back into nursing school.

Coming home from work at night, Mary would catch the Taylor bus in front of Barnes Hospital, and she got off the bus at Finney Avenue, where we live. She only had to walk two minutes to our apartment.

When Mary got off the bus every night, I watched her from my bedroom window when she passed the Sorrento Lounge on the southeast corner of Finney Avenue. I kept my eyes on her until she unlocked the front door and entered the house. I would hear her footsteps walking down the hallway, and she would enter our bedroom.

The Sorrento Cocktail Lounge and the Clover Leaf Tavern were at the corners of Taylor and Finney Avenue, across the street from one another. Those businesses were patronized by working-class labor people who went in and out of Clover Leaf Tavern; and professional and working-class office people who patronized Sorrento Cocktail Lounge.

Discounting the jovial loud voices from the "corner crowd" on the weekends, there was never any concern of safety being a question to the local residents. There was respect for the people living in the neighborhood by those patrons of the Clover Leaf Tavern and the Sorrento Lounge.

Mary did not rely on the income from her job to help support our family. Her work was more for training and reacquainting herself with the nursing environment rather than a job to earn a living.

Mary kept her commitment to Barnes Hospital and worked for six weeks. She resigned from her job and returned to Homer G. School of Nursing in August 1961.

CHAPTER 14

Mary's Junior Year—Homer G.

SINCE HE WAS BORN, FOR eight months, Mary had spent every day with Birdie, cuddling, pampering, and teaching him at 8 months, what normally a two year older would learn. Now the reality of returning to school and being separated from him during the weekdays was emotionally difficult for her.

Mary was two months shy of her twentieth birthday. I understood her being a young mother; she was emotionally torn, knowing she would be separated all week from her baby, Birdie. It was Sunday evening, and we drove to her parent's home, where Birdie would stay in East St. Louis until Friday evening.

Mary's parents were making a tremendous personal sacrifice by keeping Birdie for us. Her mother particularly had to manage their daily household with her elementary school children, and Margaret Ann was not in school yet.

Mary's parents did not charge us "one penny" to keep Birdie during the week. The money we persuaded her to take was a modest payment for babysitting their grandson. They were not keeping Birdie for pecuniary reasons but rather to help Mary and I, so she could finish nursing school.

It was time for us to leave because Mary had to report to Homer G.'s nursing dormitory tonight. Mary wanted to spend as much time as possible with Birdie before leaving him, knowing she would not see him until Friday. She was procrastinating, and Mrs. Byas said in a slightly elevated voice, "Pookie" you need to just go now. Birdie will be fine. Mary hemmed hawed around a little longer.

Mrs. Byas gave a big sigh and repeated, Pookie, go on and leave now. You are getting on my nerves; Birdie will be fine. Now that was the "Ruby Byas" tone of voice, and Mary responded quickly to her mother's demand, and we headed for the door.

Birdie was enjoying all the attention from his grandfather Byas and his young aunts, who were only three and five years older than him. He was laughing and having fun. He was comfortable at his grandparents' home and did not fuss or cry when we left the house.

Driving home, Mary solemnly expressed, "this will be Birdie's first time being away from us overnight." Responding, I assured Mary that Birdie would miss her, but he would be fine with his grandparents.

I had to take Mary to the Homer G. dormitory before her 11 pm curfew. Now I was procrastinating. I waited until the very last minute before leaving the apartment. The reality that we would be spending our nights apart was starting to sink in. Mary would stay on campus in the dormitory Sunday night through Friday evening and come home for the weekend.

Arriving at the dorm, I parked in front, and just for a moment, I had flashbacks of when Mary would ascend the steps to the dorm in her rhythmic bouncing way. Her situation was gravely different this time around. She was now a wife and a mother; this responsibility was what she had to start her junior year of nursing school with. Regardless of being away for a year, I was certain she would assimilate quickly into her effective nursing school routine again.

Mary and I had expressed our good night sentiments before we left our house. We did not want to have melancholy feelings or become emotional when we said goodnight and she entered the dormitory. We got out of the car, held hands, walking up the steps to the dormitory entrance, and said, "I love you" to one another.

This was another reality where I would kiss my wife goodnight, as she would spend her nights at the dormitory, and I would return home to spend my nights alone. I knew the first several weeks would be difficult adjusting, with Birdie staying in East St. Louis and Mary living at the nurses' dormitory during the week.

Shortly after school began, Mary quickly got **acclimated** to her school schedule. We also reestablished our previous routine from her freshman year, where we talked every night after she had her dinner. Sometimes our conversation was long; at other times, they were very short. Also, when her schedule permitted, she came home during the week, so we could see one another.

It was only natural that Mary would devote as much time and attention as possible to Birdie on the weekend. I spent my time with him as well. Often Mary didn't get much studying done on the weekends. She had adjusted to the fact that Birdie was accustomed to staying with his grandparents during the weekdays. When we picked him up, he was overly excited to see his mom on Friday evenings.

Everything was progressing very well in Mary's junior year of school. She excelled in her classes with impressive grades. She was one of the junior class leaders, as most of her classmates were basically one year removed from graduating high school.

As the calendar year was ending, I had scheduled my vacation time during Christmas week, which coincided with Mary's Christmas holiday school break. It was exciting now that Birdie had just turned one year old in November. Mary was home during Christmas week, and having our son with us was tremendous. Spending the week together as a family, celebrating Christmas with Birdie, and seeing our extended family members that week was awesome!

Before the New Year began, Mary and I had worked out our schedule where she would come home on Wednesday evening so we could spend time together. However, that arrangement created excitement and anticipation for the weekend also.

Being separated during the week and spending most of our time with Birdie on the weekends, there were times when Mary and I seemed deprived of personal time between us. It amplified some emotional moments during the short personal time we shared on weekends.

As a young normal healthy twenty-one and twenty-two years old married couple, Mary and I were deeply passionate about one another, and we had extraordinarily strong feelings and desires for each other, and we often acted like newlyweds.

However, we were also very cognizant of the fact that we both wanted Mary to finish nursing school. Therefore, Mary and I were careful in planning our time together. At times, it was personally challenging for both of us to suppress our intense feelings for one another. Consequently, our human passion, miscalculations, or whatever human factors overcame our family planning (or mis-planning).

Déjà Vu Mary Is Pregnant

Now here again, Déjà vu! Mary's junior year in nursing school was equivalent to her freshman year. She had excellent grades, enjoyed her classes, and endeavored to become a nurse. There was a difference now. She is a mother who endured not seeing her young son, "Birdie," during the weekdays. She could only physically hug and embrace him on weekends.

Mary had completed half of her junior year of nursing school when she called and asked me to come and pick her up. I was excited that she wanted to come home, especially since this was not our scheduled Wednesday for her to come home.

However, Mary did not sound enthusiastic. I was concerned and asked if everything was all right. She responded, "Let's talk when I get home."

My enthusiasm was still heightened. "Okay, baby, I will see you in a little bit."

Twenty minutes later, I was at the dormitory. Mary came down the steps and quickly got in the car. We kissed as usual; however, she was not smiling. I asked, "what do I owe this wonderful treat?" In a dry tone of voice, "Willis, we can talk when we get home, okay." My excitement was deflated slightly, and I didn't say another word driving home.

I was more curious than ever now, but I stayed cool. It took the normal twenty minutes to get home. Entering the house, Mary walked to our bedroom and stood motionless in the center of the room. Her first words were, "Willis, just hold me, please."

I put my arms around her, I didn't say anything, and I just held her tightly. Then suddenly I felt my shirt was slightly wet and I realized that Mary was crying. She then raised her head from my chest and looked me in the eyes. She said, "Willis, I am pregnant."

I paused a minute, asking, "are you sure, baby?" Her tears started flowing again. "Yes, I am positive, and I feel so embarrassed. Willis, everybody is helping us so I can finish nursing school! Now I am pregnant!" she responded. At that precise moment, I believe the weight of that responsibility was heavily on Mary's mind.

"Willis, I was conflicted when I realized that I was pregnant. This is the second time I have gotten pregnant during my nursing school career. I do not know what our families, particularly momma and Mother Drake, would feel about me being pregnant now. They have gone out of their way so I can finish nursing school," she continued.

I was hugging and trying to console Mary, telling her everything would be all right. However, I was somewhat perplexed about my feelings that she was pregnant. But first, I had to calm Mary and let her know everything would be fine.

Regaining her composure, she said, "Willis, when I realized I was pregnant, I was disappointed and saddened. The timing was just terrible for me to get pregnant. However, I still loved the idea that I was going to have another baby."

Although I, too, felt somewhat conflicted, the same way Mary did. In reality, we had a classical predicament that Mary felt was an embarrassing situation. By our behavior, unintentional as it was, our passion for one another resulted in a situation in which Mary was now pregnant. She was approaching the middle of finishing her junior year of nursing school.

I had a suppressed feeling of joy about having another baby. My other feeling was of concern because I knew the personal sacrifices that Mary had made to get to this point to finish school. I was aware of the sacrifices and expectations that her mother, specifically, and our families overall, had made so that she could finish school.

Thinking aloud, or maybe I was just mulling over in my mind the reality that we were going to have another baby. My thought process jumped to stating, "Mary, we will need our own apartment when the baby is born, regardless if you plan to go back to school or not."

During this serious in-depth conversation, Mary was calm, and she said, "Willis, I'm hungry!" I was smiling "baby, I can eat something too. Do you think this hungry thing is contagious?" We both were now laughing. I knew our situation's seriousness; we also knew everything would be okay.

Mary got up and went and opened the refrigerator. "Babe, I am gonna fix myself a Braunschweiger and Cheese sandwich. Do you want me to make you one too?" She asked. I shook my head, "yes; I want a sandwich, too," I replied. We sat at the kitchen table, ate our food, and just talked, and soon the laughter followed. Now I was confident that everything would work out just fine.

Time passed quickly, and it was time to take Mary back to the dorm. Driving there, we continued talking about "what-if situations." After we talked, I knew the problem did not seem that monumental anymore. We knew everything would be okay, as we just trusted in the Lord God Almighty.

Mary was smiling when we got to the dormitory. The heavy burden seemed to be lifted from her. I kissed her and assured her that all was well. "Willis, regardless of what it is, you always let me know everything will be all right. Baby, I love you, and thank you for loving me," she concluded, feeling confident.

I sat in the car, watching Mary go up the steps as she entered the dormitory. I drove off, and when I got home, I called to ensure she was still feeling okay.

Announcing to Our Family That Mary Was Expecting
On Friday evening, I picked Mary up from school as usual. Normally we would go straight to East St. Louis to pick up Birdie. We had talked earlier, and Mary wanted to tell our parents that she was pregnant this weekend. She decided it would be convenient to stop at mother's house first and tell her she was pregnant. Then we would go to pick up Birdie and tell her parents the news.

Under normal circumstances, notwithstanding the fact that Mary was hoping to finish nursing school first, this would have been great news to share with our parents. They would have been overjoyed to hear that we were going to have another baby. However, both of our parents were hoping that Mary would finish nursing school before we had another child.

Mary said I want to tell Mother Drake as soon as possible because she thought mother might already know she is pregnant. The Holy Spirit had never failed to let mother know when one of her daughters or daughters-in-law was pregnant. In my family, it was a proven fact that any time mother had this vision of handling fish, one of her daughters or a daughter-in-law was going to have a baby. Mother would know before either her daughter or daughter-in-law knew she was pregnant.

"Willis, Mother Drake has done everything she could to help me get through nursing school. Now I am pregnant," said Mary. I know both of our parents will be disappointed." We were at mother's house, and Mary was apparently nervous about how to tell her the news. As we walked up the steps and entered the house, Mary said, "Willis, I will just tell Mother Drake straight-out that I am expecting."

Trying to be supportive, I agreed that is the best way to let her know. Mother heard us come into the house, and she called out, "Hi, is that you, Willis? Is Mary with you?" She was now in the family room, saying, "Mary, it is so good to see you. How are you doing, baby," she reached out and hugged Mary, holding her longer than usual and patting her on her back.

Mother, now holding Mary's hands and at arm's length, looking at her, said, "Mary, you look a little tired. Let's sit down on the couch and tell me how school was going." Sitting side-by-side on the couch, they were laughing and chitchatting, and mother seemed to enjoy having time to catch up with Mary on her school. I was sitting on the second step of the stairwell, where I usually sat when I came with Mary to visit my parents.

We had been at the house for fifteen minutes. Mary had avoided, or at least prolonged, the reason we had come to talk to mother. I told Mary we still had to go to East St. Louis to pick up Birdie and we should get started.

Now Mary was not looking directly at mother. Then she said, "Mother Drake, I have something I need to tell you; I am pregnant." Tears had welled up in Mary's eyes. Mother smiled as she put her arms around Mary's shoulders, pulling her closer and hugging her.

Mother had a smile on her face as she said, "Yes, Mary, I already knew you were pregnant, and you are going to have a baby girl." I had a vision three weeks ago, and I knew you were the one pregnant.

Mother was still hugging Mary, and she raised Mary's head so she could see her eyes. "Mary, it was revealed to me three times that you will finish nursing school too, and you will be a wonderful nurse."

I think those words of encouragement alone, coming from mother, lifted Mary's spirit because she knew that mother's visions if confirmed three times, would always come true. Mary seemed more composed now. Then she said, "Mother Drake, I hope you are not too disappointed that I am pregnant."

Mother's smile now turned into light laughter. She said, "Mary, I cannot wait to take care of that baby girl when you are back in nursing school."

We left mother's house, driving over to East St. Louis to pick up Birdie and to tell Mary's mother that she is pregnant. In short order, we were at Mary's parents' home.

We went into the house, and Mary immediately called, "Birdie, Birdie, it's momma baby." Hearing his mother's voice, Birdie came toddling towards her. Mary swooped him up in her arms and hugged and kissed him. Mary absorbed all the love from her baby Birdie. Then I took him from Mary and gave him his imaginary airplane ride, tossing him in the air.

Mary hugged her mother in the living room. She said hi to her dad. He greeted Mary and I and said, "Birdie, that grandson of mine is moving all over this house." While I was holding Birdie in my arms, Mr. Byas tickled his stomach, and he just laughed.

Finally, things settled down after Mary had seen Birdie, her sisters, and her brothers. Now the kids had returned to their room, and Mary sat on the couch next to her mother. Her dad was still standing in the middle of the living room, as I was also.

Mary did not beat around the bush. She said, "Momma, I am pregnant; we are going to have a baby." Mrs. Byas had a subdued look on her face, and she said, "Pookie, when is the baby due?" She hugged Mary and injected her humor, telling Mary, "Pookie, now two children are enough."

I couldn't tell initially from Mrs. Byas' facial expression if perhaps she had mixed emotions or was slightly disappointed or not. She knew how much Mary wanted to finish nursing school and become a nurse. Mr. Byas had a beaming smile on his face, although he didn't say a word. I think his smile spoke volumes without him opening his mouth. He was going to have another grandchild.

Then like a crescendo echoing in the room, Mary said, "Momma, when I told Mother Drake that I was pregnant, she said, "she had a vision three weeks ago that revealed I was pregnant with a baby girl. She also told me that I would finish nursing school." Mrs. Byas also had learned of my mother's gift of having true visions, and when confirmed, they would always be true.

It was in April 1962 when Mary knew she was expecting (pregnant). She had only three months remaining, and there was no problem with her finishing her second (junior) year of nursing school. She had excellent grades.

Mary's Second Pregnancy
However, Mary would not be able to enroll in nursing school that coming August to complete her senior and final year of school. She was mostly concerned if she would be able to enroll the following year as a senior in the Homer G. nursing school to finish nursing school.

From a practical and realistic situation, Mary and I could not think too far into the future. We had to focus on our immediate issues and concerns. The reality was that we were going to have our second child in 1962.

We would now have additional expenses to raise our family with a new baby on the way. Therefore, it was a long leap that we had to get to before we had to address Mary enrolling back in the Homer G. Nursing School for her senior year.

I do not recall being nervous or apprehensive about having a new baby. I had faith that everything was going to be fine. Ma Dear would always say, "Just trust in Lord God Almighty." The immediate concern was how we were going to take care of a new baby in our family."

Mary Finished Her Junior Year of Nursing School
Academically, Mary had a successful junior year at school despite her dual roles as a student, mother, and wife. She had completed the school year managing all three responsibilities exceptionally well.

At the end of her school year, I picked Mary up at the dorm, and she was content as she got in the car. I asked comically, "why are you so joyous this evening?" She said, "Willis, I had my year-end conversation (review) with Miss. Gore this afternoon, and she gave me my grade assessment; she let me know 'that I had achieved excellent grades in all of my classes and my clinical work in the hospital wards was done very well also.'"

Mary said, "Willis, what made me the happiest? It surprised me when Miss. Gore asked, "if I was planning to return to school after my baby was born to complete my training to be a registered nurse?"

Mary said she conveyed strongly to Miss. Gore, "Yes, ma'am, I most certainly plan to return to school after my baby is born. I am "determined" to be a registered nurse. Miss. Gore, I sincerely appreciate you giving me the opportunity to complete my nursing training at Homer G. The burning desire within me is proof that I am destined to be a registered nurse.

"Willis, uncharacteristically, Miss Gore gave me a tight hug and said, "Mrs. Drake, I look forward to you returning to finish your nursing training at Homer G., and I just know you are going to be a terrific nurse one day."

As Mary completed her second year of nursing training, there was only one rung on the proverbial ladder to climb. She would be absent during the next school year and prepare to have our second child.

Mary was now transiting from being a full-time second-year junior nursing student to again being a full-time bonafide mom, expecting a new baby in five months. She was getting everything arranged with her pediatrician, Doctor Homer Nash, and continuing the experience of being a wife, mother, and homemaker.

Instead of having to hit the nursing books in the classroom, she was now teaching her son "Birdie" his basic skills, ABCs, numbers, counting, and the normal skills a one-year-old baby should be learning, and more complex things as well.

CHAPTER 15

Birth of Monica

D URING THE EARLY STAGES OF her pregnancy, Mary didn't have any particular food cravings. However, in the latter stages, she had a unique craving for crushed ice cubes or small ice chips. Whenever she got the urge, she would suck the ice chips day and night.

Based on "Mother's confirmed vision, Mary was convinced that she was having a baby girl, and she was buying baby clothes for a girl. She was prepping Birdie for having a baby sister, and being a big brother was especially important. Week by week, Birdie was getting excited for his new baby sister to be born.

Two weeks before her delivery date, Mary packed a suitcase with a pink baby outfit and blanket she would need to bring our baby home from the hospital. A week later, I was sound asleep at 3:30 in the early morning, and Mary called my name twice.

"Willis, Willis," I woke up, and she said, "I am ready to go to the hospital!" Get my suitcase and help me get ready. I jumped out of bed, and I was cool, and I didn't get excited. I helped Mary to get up and get dressed. I called out for Tee and told her Mary was ready to go to the hospital."

A few minutes later, Tee rushed into our bedroom and asked Mary, "how close are your contractions?" With a frown on her face and her hand on her stomach, Mary said, "I am not sure, maybe 15 or 20 minutes apart, Tee."

Willis, hurry up and get Mary to the hospital. At that moment, Birdie woke up, and I told him, "Mommy is going to the hospital to have your baby sister." Tee said, "Willis, go on, and I will take care of Birdie." Mary was holding my arm as we walked to the front door.

Mary appeared calm as we left the house, and I drove to Firmin Desloge Hospital. We had a sporadic conversation, mostly me asking how she was feeling. When we arrived at the hospital, the registration process was efficient, and Mary was quickly admitted to the maternity delivery ward.

Contrary to her first delivery, Mary was in labor for a brief time, and she had a relatively easy delivery giving birth to our baby girl, who was born at 7:29 am Monday, December 17, 1962. We named her Monica Renee Drake.

A few days after Monica was born, Mary was up and moving around the hospital's maternity ward. Her recovery was on schedule, and she was discharged Thursday morning, three days after giving birth to Monica. I got to the hospital at 10:00 o'clock. Mary and Monica both were dressed and ready when I arrived in the room. Monica was sound asleep in Mary's arms, wrapped in her pink baby blanket.

It was a cold December day. We left the hospital and arrived home, I got out of the car and took Monica in my arms, and I helped Mary up the steps to our apartment.

Tee opened the front door, and she reached to take Monica from my arms. The smile on Tee's face was revealing as she carefully caressed Monica in her arms and carried her to our bedroom. She whispered, "Birdie is asleep as Mary and I walked into the bedroom.

Tee placed Monica in her bassinet and asked Mary if she was feeling okay. "I feel pretty good, Tee, but I think I will lie-down and rest a minute. Tee tell me, how does Monica look to you?" Tee was beaming as her face lit up, saying in her very expressive ways. "Mary, she is adorable, just a beautiful baby."

I know Bill (my mother's nickname) is going to be crazy about her. I think Monica kind of favors Bill also. They both laughed quietly as Mary slowly stood up and looked in the bassinet, smiling down at Monica.

Looking at Mary beaming upon Monica, I could tell she realized how much joy the birth of Monica had instantly brought to our family. Mary sat back down in the chair with a satisfying smile on her face.

Birdie started stirring, waking up, and Mary said, "Tee, I can't wait to see Birdie's reaction when he first sees his baby sister."

Birdie was awake now, standing up in his baby crib, asking, "Momma, my baby sister home?" We laughed, and he was excited to see his "little baby sister." He reached up for me to lift him out of his baby crib. I held him high so he could "see his little baby sister sleeping in her bassinet."

Mary immediately embraced Birdie in her arms, hugging him; she said, "you haven't seen me in four days; give momma a kiss. I know you are happy to see your baby sister, but we will have to be quiet, so we don't wake her up, okay? Her name is Monica. Can you say "Monica?" Birdie, with a smile on his face, said, "Monica."

As Mary got in bed, jokingly, I said, with Monica's bassinet in our bedroom, it reminds me of when Charles, Kermit Jr., Melvin, and I shared this same bedroom. Baby, when your parents come to see Monica, it's going to be crowded in this room. Mary said it would be okay; we would have our own apartment soon.

Mrs. Byas had seen Monica at the hospital, albeit she was separated by the glass partition in the baby nursery. Mary's parents were coming this weekend to see their granddaughter, Monica. This would be Mr. Byas' first time seeing her.

Saturday afternoon, Mr. and Mrs. Byas arrived at our apartment to welcome their granddaughter Monica to the Byas family. Mrs. Byas smiled from ear to ear as she held Monica in her arms. We were in the crowded bedroom, but that did not matter. The excitement and attention, rightly so, were focused on "Monica."

However, Birdie was not being slighted. He was sitting on his granddad's lap, who was giving him plenty of attention as he always did. After several hours, when Mary's parents were ready to leave, I walked with them to the front door. We hugged and shook hands, and I thanked them for coming to see Mary and their granddaughter, Monica.

I returned to the bedroom, and Mary was beaming with joy that her parents had come to see and bless their granddaughter. I put the chairs back in the kitchen, and suddenly the bedroom seemed a little larger. Mary now had Monica in the bed with her, and she was goo talking to her, and I was sitting in the chair holding Birdie on my lap.

CHAPTER 16

Our First Apartment— 3715 Fair Avenue

W

HEN MARY WAS SIX MONTHS pregnant, it was apparent that we would need our own apartment after the baby was born. December arrived seemingly so rapidly, and Monica was born. The reality of needing our own apartment was magnified after we brought Monica home from the hospital. With Monica's bassinet now in the bedroom, our living quarters suddenly felt cramped, with us basically living in a single bedroom.

The next week we celebrated our first Christmas with Willis Jr. and Monica. Then the New Year was on the horizon. I told Mary we would let Tee know that we would be looking to get our own apartment soon after the first of the New Year.

Monica was ten weeks old, and the weather was turning milder, and it was ideal to start looking for an apartment. Tee, always the rational person, said, "oh, you kids, I knew this day was coming soon. Most certainly, having two children, you will need your own apartment now."

I had never looked for an apartment to rent before. So every weekend, I checked the classified advertisement section of the Sunday's St. Louis Post Dispatch Newspaper, looking for apartments for rent.

The third weekend looking, I saw an "ad" for a four-room apartment for rent. Of all the ads I had looked at previously, this particular ad caught my eye. It was nothing different or unusual about the listing, but it attracted my attention for some reason.

The apartment was located in North St. Louis, and I vacillated about going to see it. Then impulsively, I told Mary, "I saw an apartment for rent in the newspaper that I was going to check out." She was feeding Monica, glanced at me, and said, "okay, I will see you when you get back."

The apartment was located at 3715 Fair Avenue near the corner of Fair and Natural Bridge Avenues. It would take me twenty-five minutes to drive there. The "newspaper Ad" stated to ring the tenant's doorbell across from the vacant apartment, and they would show the apartment to prospective renters.

I was not so familiar with this North St. Louis neighborhood. When I attended Sumner High School, I was familiar with "Ivy's Snack Shop" on Lambdin Avenue, which had the best fish sandwiches. I drove across Newstead Avenue to Kennerly Avenue (two blocks from Homer G.) and turned left on Lambdin Avenue, and then the street name changed to Fair Avenue.

As soon as I crossed Natural Bridge, there was a Standard Oil "Service (filling) Station" on the northwest corner at Fair and Natural Bridge Avenues. An alleyway separated the filling station from the apartment buildings in the 3700 block of Fair Ave. There were three very well-kept four-family apartment buildings next to one another there on the block.

The apartment building at 3715 Fair Avenue was a red brick building, and the door to enter the building was light brown with two vertical glass panes in the door. There was a small vestibule with a marble floor where the mailbox and doorbell for each apartment unit were located. The outside door was always unlocked to allow the United States Postman to deliver the mail.

There was one apartment on the South side and one on the north side of the building, on both the first and second levels. I rang the doorbell of the person living in the apartment across from the vacant apartment.

A man in his mid-sixties answered the door. He gave me the "twice look-over" as if he was going to decide if I could rent the apartment. Being very congenial, I said, "Good morning, and introduced myself. I asked to look at the vacant apartment for rent."

I do not recall the man's name now, but he was polite and introduced himself. He let me into the vacant apartment. He stood outside in the hallway and said, "When you're finished looking at the apartment, let me know when you leave."

I looked through the apartment thoroughly in fifteen minutes and was convinced this apartment was ideal for our family. It was unfurnished, with two bedrooms, a living room, an average size kitchen, and a bathroom. The apartment was clean, with a central heating system, but there was no air-conditioning.

When I was ready to leave, I thanked the man and asked how I could contact the owner to rent the apartment. He said Mrs. Barnes was the owner, and he gave me her telephone number.

He asked if I had children. I told him like a proud father, "Yes, sir; I have two young children. He said without hesitating, "I do not think Mrs. Barnes will rent the apartment to anyone with children." Sir, are you sure. He repeated himself, "yes, that is what she told me." I thanked him for showing me the apartment, and I left feeling disappointed.

For the 25 minutes driving home, I felt dispirited. I thought when I first walked into that apartment, I felt in my spirit that this "apartment" was suited for our family. I was now agonizing over the idea that the owner would not rent to anyone with children.

The apartment was fifteen minutes from Homer G., which would be convenient when Mary returned to nursing school. It was in a safe and comfortable neighborhood, and Fairgrounds Park was across the street. However, I would have to tell Mary, "The owner would not rent to anyone with children."

When I entered the house, Tee called out from her bedroom, "Willis, did you like the apartment?" In a dry tone, "Yes, Tee, I really like the apartment, but the owner will not rent to people with children." Tee emerged from her room and displayed her optimistic attitude, "Willis, don't worry; I'm sure you will find the right apartment soon."

I went into our bedroom and told Mary how much I liked the apartment, but the owner would not rent to people with children. Babe, "for some reason, my inner spirit was compelling me to call and talk directly to the owner, Mrs. Barnes." Mary said, "Willis when you have those strong feelings, normally that means something positive will happen. You should just call and talk to her."

Mary's positive attitude quickly convinced me to call Mrs. Barnes. The phone rang twice, and I heard a lady's voice say hello. Responding rapidly, "Hello, may I please speak with Mrs. Barnes? She said in a firm voice, "yes, I am Mrs. Barnes; how can I help you?"

I told her my name and that I had looked at the apartment, located at 3715 Fair Ave., and my wife and I would like to rent the apartment. We have a two-year-old son and a four-month-old daughter. She interrupted me and said, "I am sorry, Mr. Drake, but I just don't want to rent the apartment to anyone with children."

In the next breath, I asked, "If I could come and talk with her in person?" She was hesitant at first, but she acquiesced and gave me her home address, and I could come to see her now. She lived on Highland Avenue, east of Kingshighway, in either the 4800 or 4900 block.

In twenty minutes, I was at Mrs. Barnes' house. She lived in an upstairs unit of a two-family duplex building that she owned. I rang the doorbell, and I had a very positive feeling that meeting me, she would be convinced to rent the apartment to me. Mrs. Barnes opened the door relatively quickly, and it was apparent that she was expecting me. She invited me into the house, and we walked to the top of the stairs, and we stood at the doorway entrance and talked.

I assured Mrs. Barnes, "I give you my word; if you rent the apartment to me, I promise to treat it as my personal home." She said, "Mr. Drake, there is something about you, and I cannot explain it, but I can tell you are a fine young man." Her voice was low as she said, "something touched my heart, and I am going to take a chance to rent the apartment to you."

I thanked Mrs. Barnes, and I assured her that my wife and I would take care of the apartment and I would pay my rent on time every month. I was only at Mrs. Barnes' house for fifteen minutes, and my prayer was answered. I know that's why Mrs. Barnes rented me the apartment.

When I returned home, I had a smile on my face, and both Mary and Tee knew, without me saying a word, that I was able to rent the apartment. I hugged Mary and whispered in her ear, "we got the apartment." Mrs. Barnes said, "after she saw and talked with me, something changed her heart about renting me the apartment."

I asked Tee if she would watch the kids, so I could take Mary to see the apartment. Mary was excited, and she got dressed quickly, and we went to go see the apartment. When we got to Kennerly and Lambdin Avenues, Mary said, "Homer G. is only a few blocks from here.

That will be convenient living so close to Homer G." It was only a few minutes until we crossed Natural Bridge, and I made a U-turn and parked in front of the apartment building that displayed 3715 above the door.

I rang the tenant's doorbell and asked if my wife could please see the apartment. He let us in the apartment and said, "when you are finished looking at the apartment, please just close and lock the door when you leave."

Mary entered the apartment in front of me, and I was intentionally silent. I wanted her to look at the apartment without my influence regarding whether she liked the apartment or not. I observed Mary's body language, particularly her facial expressions, as she walked through the apartment. From her overall expression, I could tell that she was pleased with the apartment.

Hardwood floors were in the living room and front and back bedrooms. The kitchen had an attractive linoleum-covered floor. The bathroom had a white marble patterned floor design. There was a back door in the back bedroom, which would be Birdie's and Monica's bedroom. The door leads to a back porch or a finished enclosed sunroom.

We could use the room in the summertime to sit in or for an area where the kids could play instead of going outside to play in the fenced backyard.

Mary had made her full assessment of the apartment, and I saw that smile on her face as she said, "yea, babe, I like this apartment. Now we just have to get the furniture we need, so I can make this apartment truly become our home."

Standing in the vacant apartment, I was pleased that Mary was satisfied. I was delivering on my promise to my wife that I would get us our own apartment, and we would purchase furniture for the apartment that she would be satisfied with.

We left the apartment, and driving home, I told Mary we needed to finalize our rental agreement with Mrs. Barnes first, and then we could plan to purchase the furniture we needed. We returned home, and Tee was sitting on the couch in the living room, holding Monica. Birdie was sitting on the floor in front of her, playing.

Before I could close the door, Tee said, "well, Mary, do you like the apartment?" Mary sat on the couch next to Tee and started describing the apartment. I called Mrs. Barnes to let her know my wife likes the apartment, and I want to come to pay the rent and get the keys so we can move into the apartment as soon as possible.

Routinely, Mary and I would visit our parents' homes every Sunday. As a young couple, we still indirectly sought our parents' advice before we made major decisions. It was automatic that we would inform our parents that we had found an apartment to rent and would be moving shortly. Also, we had to purchase furniture for the apartment."

Leaving my parents' house, we went to East St. Louis to share with Mary's parents that we had rented our own apartment and would be moving next week. It was apparent that our parents were proud that we were getting our own apartment and could pay cash for the furniture to totally furnish the apartment.

On Tuesday evening, when the stores stayed open until 9:00 pm, we would shop at the Lambert's Furniture Store at 911 Washington Ave. That store was considered the high-end furniture store in the St. Louis city area at that time.

Professional and upper-income people purchased furniture at Lambert's. I recall Mrs. Mae Layne (Dr. Richard Layne's wife) telling me when I was a young kid working for her, "Drake, if you want good furniture, buy it at Lambert's Furniture Store in downtown St. Louis."

That Tuesday evening, mother kept the kids while Mary and I went to Lambert's to purchase our furniture. I deferred to Mary's judgment to select the furniture she wanted as long as she stayed within our budget. Mary basically knew what she wanted, and she only had to decide on the particular style, color, and nuances of the furniture she needed to purchase.

Smiling, she said, "Willis, you know I am not an extravagant person, and I will shop for the best bargains possible. I am going to make the apartment into our home; you just wait and see." I told Mary, "as long as I have a place for my High-Fidelity (Hi-Fi) Stereo System, I will be fine." Laughing, she said, "Willis, that style of mahogany color furniture isn't made anymore. I do not want anything clashing with my color scheme." Mary knew my Hi-Fi system would be part of our furniture regardless.

We were in the store for five minutes, and a salesman approached us, introduced himself, and gave us his salesman's card. He asked if he could help us find anything. I told him we knew what we wanted to purchase. However, we needed more detailed information about the Italian couches that were on sale.

He escorted us to the area where the Italian couches were on display. Suddenly, Mary stopped in front of this one couch and said emphatically, "Willis, this is the couch I want. It is the exact light blue color fabric and everything I envisioned." My concern was the price tag, and I said, "Mary, the price of this couch is what we would pay for the entire living room furniture."

The salesman cautiously spoke up and said, "Mrs. Drake, you have a good eye for furniture. That is an excellent couch, and it is on sale at a considerably reduced price by forty percent off." Now I felt more comfortable, knowing we could afford the actual sale price within our budget. Plus, Mary was going to be satisfied too.

There was a storewide sale that evening, and Mary was able to purchase all the furniture she wanted within our budget. After Mary had selected the couch she wanted, selecting the remaining living room furniture fell right in place. She selected the chair, two end tables, table lamps, and a matching coffee table.

For the kitchen furniture and appliances, Mary selected a Coppertone color cooking stove and refrigerator and a brownish dinette table and chair-set that she liked. She also was able to purchase her silverware, table place settings, cooking pots, and pans as well. She purchased a three-piece bedroom suite with a full-size bed, a dresser with a mirror, and a chest of drawers.

Observing Mary, I could tell she was satisfied and happy. We had purchased all the furniture except a chest of drawers and a toy chest for Birdie's and Monica's room. We signed the necessary paperwork, paid for the merchandise we had purchased and were given a delivery scheduled for Friday morning.

We went to pick up the kids. Mary naturally had to give mother the details of the furniture we bought, especially the deal we got on the Italian-style couch.

Returning home, we settled into our normal nightly routine. The next day, time was moving along very quickly, and Mary and I had two days to clean the apartment to her standards. With minimum effort, we spruced up the apartment on Thursday evening and were ready for the furniture to be delivered on Friday.

The Lambert deliverymen arrived on schedule Friday; and placed the furniture in the apartment without a scratch. We took our personal belongings to our apartment, and on Saturday morning, Mary, Birdie, Monica, and I moved into our apartment. Mary was able to put the final decorative touches on the apartment, and it was now our home.

Mary was home with Willis Jr. and Monica in her role as a young mother. When I got home from work, we would have dinner as a family, and I would share time with the kids until their bedtime.

We were now living in our own apartment. So it felt great to come home from work and, figuratively speaking, have my wife meet me at the door with the kids in tow. I knew this situation would change in several months when Mary returned to nursing school. She now had five months before she would become a student again at Homer G Phillips nursing school. This would be her senior and final year of school.

Mary had her daily routine set. She would get Birdie and Monica up and dressed and fix their breakfast at the same time every morning. She also had their naps scheduled at a specified time in the afternoon each day. She was training them now for the time when she would return to nursing school later in the year.

Mary often discussed finishing the final year of nursing school. Joking, I would tell her, "you have learned to "Burn really well in the kitchen," and I will miss those good home-cooked meals when you are back in nursing school."

136

Mary would say, "well, just think of what you have to look forward to on the weekends when I'm home." Looking straight into her eyes when you come home, "Baby, you can bet your cooking is not what I will be looking forward to the most on the weekend!" We both would just fall out laughing, cracking up.

CHAPTER 17

◇

Mary's Final Year—
Homer G. Nursing School

◇

W E SETTLED INTO OUR APARTMENT comfortably, and our family was getting adjusted to a new community. There were three senior couples living in the apartment building. Two were African-Americans, and one was a white couple. There were no children living in the apartment building.

In this new residential environment, instead of being five minutes away from my parent's home, we now lived twenty-five minutes from them. However, we could walk across the street to the Fairgrounds Community Park, Natural Bridge, and Fair Avenues. The park extended east, down to North Grand Avenue, and extended north over to Kossuth street.

The trees started to blossom as the weather started getting warmer, and in the mornings, I could hear the birds chirping. These were signs that the spring of the year was upon us. Within only weeks, the warm weather had fully arrived, and in the evenings, after eating dinner, I would take Willis Jr. to Fairgrounds Park to play. At two years old, he was just getting confidence in running without the fear of falling.

He would run, and I pretended that I couldn't catch him. I would let him play until he was tuckered out. Then we would go home, and back in the apartment, I would cuddle and play with Monica. Later I would bathe Willis Jr.; Mary would read him a bedtime story and put the kids to bed.

For the most part, this was our routine each evening. My interaction with the kids allowed Mary to mentally escape from her role as a mother for a brief time. Mary had not started her study routine to return to nursing school. She had four months, until mid-August, before returning for her final year at Homer G. nursing school.

Her focus now was to spend time with the kids, and as she would say, "Willis, I want to store up some love" for when I am back at school in August. I know I will miss my two little "munchkins" so much.

Miss. Gore had already assured Mary's return to finish her final year at Homer G. Putting Mary's total nursing school experience in perspective, I marveled at how she was so blessed, destined, and determined. She was also motivated and dedicated to being a nurse.

Initially, in the 1959–1960 class school years, Mary started her Homer G. student nursing career, and she would have been a member of the Homer G. 1962 graduating class. However, Mary persevered and was now getting ready to start her senior year as a member of the Homer G. nursing school graduating class of 1964.

There were 29 student nurses in her 1959–1960 class, the year she entered HGP nursing school. Mary was one of only three students who did not finish that class. Twenty-six of the 29 students in that class graduated in 1962: Grace B. Adams, Evelyn E. Allen, Vernell Brooks, Murray G. Brown, Corrine Clemons, Annie S. Crawford, Hilderd Cromartie, Esther C. Darris, Anna P. Davis, Constance M. Fitzpatrick, Delores Graham, Doris S. Hurvey, Florence M. Matthews, Dorenda McClain, Coldova McGlaun, Bobbie J. Miller, Sandra Nelson, Ressie M. Parram, Floydie A. Scott, Havolyn D. Scott, Marva Shegog, Loretta Stewart, Lenette Torian, Florence G. Washington, Dorothy Wilson, Selma U. Woods.

Overall, Mary overcame becoming a mother twice in her first two years of nursing school. This could have crushed the average young woman's dreams. However, nothing would cause Mary to give up on her becoming a nurse. At this point, the normal possibility of her completing nursing school following her freshman year was highly questionable. Again, but for the "grace of God, this was not possible."

Mary's Senior Year of Nursing School

The dawn of Mary's senior year of nursing school had finally arrived. The reality that she would be away from her children the entire week would be again stressful for her. However, she had laid the groundwork so Birdie and Monica were prepared and would understand the situation.

We left the apartment, Mary had her suitcase in hand, and Birdie, Monica, and I were in the car driving her to the Homer G. Nurses dormitory. She was semi-emotional, considering that she had to live at the Homer G. dormitory from 11:00 0'clock Sunday night until 4:30 pm Friday.

When we arrived at the dormitory, Mary hugged and kissed Birdie and Monica. However, she kept her composure, so the kids will not start crying. Quickly she gave them a final embrace and instantly exited the car, ascended the steps, and entered the dorm.

With Mary now a resident student nurse at Homer G., I headed home to experience my first night alone as a dad taking care of Birdie and Monica. Mary knew the sacrifice being made now would be beneficial overall, and it was part of her life's spiritual journey.

Mary had stipulated exactly how I should get the kids ready for bed at night and up in the mornings, get them dressed, and fix their breakfast. Now living less than 15 minutes from the Homer G. nursing school, depending on Mary's school schedule, I could pick her up sometimes so she could "come home to see the kids" during the week.

On my way to work, I would drop the kids at mother's house. She babysat Birdie and Monica and her grandson Wayne Gooch and granddaughter "little Shirley" (Shirley Drake-Hairston), who lived with mother. I would pick the kids up in the evenings after work.

When Mary was home on the weekends, she would prepare food for our dinner during the week. When we got home from mother's house each evening, I only had to warm up the meal we would eat for dinner.

After dinner, I would call Mary and let the kids talk to her. It was obvious that just hearing their voices each night lifted Mary's spirits tremendously. Most evenings, I would take Monica and Birdie to Fairgrounds Park. I would push Monica in her stroller while Birdie would run and play in the park. After returning home, I would bathe and put them to bed.

That was our routine, and as the summer months rolled into the fall and winter, we became housebound. Birdie and Monica had plenty of toys to play with; Mary had bought them storybooks, and I would read bedtime stories to them.

During Mary's Christmas school break was when we had the most fun together as a family. Mary had wrapped presents for the kids, and celebrating Christmas was a special time for our family. The joy of Mary seeing Birdie and Monica opening their Christmas presents, and playing with their toys, seemed to reinvigorate her.

When she returns to school, she can reflect on her good memories of seeing her two little munchkins during Christmas break.

Effectively, as the New Year had begun, we were sequestered inside the apartment, surviving the winter weather. However, time seemed to accelerate through the winter months, and springtime was breaking through the cold weather. Mary was now in the "home stretch," to use a baseball metaphor, of finishing her senior year of school.

Nursing Training at St. Louis City Hospital Number 1
To complete their registered nurses' program requirements, the Homer G. nursing students had to live at the South St. Louis City Hospital (# 1) student nurses' campus facility for three weeks. There were two situations that had an impact on her. One incident was disappointing, and the other one was influential.

During her three weeks of residency at the South St Louis City hospital (# 1), Mary experienced the theft of her favorite "yellow dress." She did her laundry one evening, washing, and drying her clothes in the nurses' laundry room. However, to prevent her dress from getting so wrinkled in the dryer, she hung the dress on a clothesline in the laundry room to dry.

When she returned to get her clothes, her dress was missing from the clothesline. She assumed with certainty that one of the South St Louis City hospital student nurses had pilfered her dress. Conversely, Mary never had a single item stolen during her two and a half years as a resident student nurse living in the Homer G. dormitory.

The theft of her dress unsettled her. "The idea that there is no trustworthiness among some of the white student nurses was very disappointing. Willis, right now, I am disturbed about this situation. That was the first dress you had bought for me, and I adored it," she complained.

Also, as part of the nurses' training, they had to observe live court cases being tried in the St. Louis City Circuit Court. Mary's court monitoring experience occurred during her final week of training; while residing at the South St Louis City hospital student nurses' dorm. Her court experience was more influential, and subsequently, it indirectly impacted her nursing career.

Mary came home Friday evening excited to be finished with that nursing requirement and glad to be back at her Homer G. nursing environment. However, she was slouched on the couch with Birdie and Monica on either side, excited to see her family. The kids hugged their mom and went to wash up for dinner.

Still seated on the couch, Mary proceeded to describe this interesting criminal court case she had observed this week. I was surprised at how animated she described the defense attorney's strategy in defending his client. She said, "that attorney made me think of the lawyers on TV. He was exceptional in unraveling the prosecutor's witnesses' testimonies. I don't recall his name, but I remember his summation was excellent. The jury returned in 30 minutes with a not guilty verdict."

Now smiling, Mary asked if dinner was ready, and we went to the kitchen and engaged the kids about their day, and we had our usual evening routine. Mary talked about getting back to the rigor of HGP nursing after spending three weeks at the South St Louis City hospital nursing campus.

A week after completing her training at the South St Louis City campus and returning to the HGP environment, Mary came into the house in complete jubilation. "Willis, guess what. Beginning next week, I will no longer have to live in the HGP dormitory." I embraced her tightly in my arms, saying, "Baby, are you sure, baby!"

She was grinning like a Cheshire cat. Yes, yes, I am sure. As a senior married student, I will be able to come home at 4:30 in the evening and stay home at night. I will report to the nurse's dorm at 7:30 in the morning for my classes and hospital clinical assignments.

With this tremendous change in her living accommodations, our family would again function more traditionally. Birdie and Monica were ecstatic every evening when I picked up their mom from the HGP dorm on our way home.

On Mary's part, she could now envision the light at the end of the proverbial tunnel. Getting in the car, she would shout out, "Only have 10 more weeks to go." At this point, she was in an exhilarating countdown mode, and the kids would crack up.

Mary being home every night was particularly great for the kids and me too. After we got home in the evenings, Mary, the kids, and I would walk in Fairgrounds Park for an hour or so. At the age of two, Monica did not like to walk. So Mary would push her in her stroller as Birdie, Mary and I walked in the park.

The countdown, week by week, continued. Mary was now inching closer to her graduation and her dream of becoming a registered nurse. Often I would tell her, "you didn't let any postponements or inconveniences alter your desire to become a nurse! You stayed true to your spiritual calling and displayed the everlasting desire that was the "Holy Spirit's gift to you."

I observed how she had sacrificed to become a registered nurse. I was in awe of the dedication and faithfulness she demonstrated along her journey. Over the five years she was in nursing school, the Holy Spirit touched her life and provided her with what she needed to become a "nurse" at each turn in her journey.

I could tell that Mary's inter-spirit had been cultivated, which made it possible, through God's grace, that her desire to become a nurse would be fulfilled. In my eyesight, "She was "destined and determined!"

I am steadfast in the belief that without being blessed, Mary becoming a registered nurse never could have happened! I sincerely believe Mary and I were "equally yoked," and it was manifested in our lives and commitment to one another's hopes, dreams, and aspirations.

Without Mary's parent's sacrifices, her becoming a nurse would not have been possible. Their support, since she was a child, was paramount in Mary becoming the person she became, and most certainly in her becoming a registered nurse.

CHAPTER 18

◇

Mary Graduates—
Homer G. Nursing School

◇

EXCEPT FOR THE BIRTH OF our two children, Mary's graduation accomplishment at the time was the most important achievement we shared as a family. With the opportunity, her tenacity, and the grace of God, Mary fulfilled her dream and destiny to become a Registered Nurse.

She persevered for five years to complete the three-year accredited diploma nursing school program. With the presumed unprecedented opportunity provided by Miss. Minnie Edythe T. Gore, for Mary to continue in the HGP Nursing School Program, she would not be denied under any circumstance. She was destined and determined!

Mary said with excitement on the evening of her graduation, "Willis, the demanding schoolwork and heavy lifting is over now, babe, as she gave a sigh." She appeared calm as she got dressed for her graduation ceremony. Laughing as she turned her back to me and asked if I would button up her uniform.

Then she put her nurse's cap on her head and used hairpins to secure it. She displayed with vivaciousness, saying, "when I am walking across the stage to receive my diploma, it will be a piece of cake." Then she laughed softly, looking at her two little munchkins.

Birdie told his mother how pretty she looked in her nurse uniform. Monica was underfoot, wanting to dress up too. It was now 6:00 pm, and Mary had finished dressing. Her uniform fitted her very well, and she looked stunning with her white apron and her nurse's cap on her head.

It was not only the uniform that made her look so regal and professional. Moreso, I could see the pride in her face and the joy in her demeanor, knowing she had prevailed over the two wonderful blessings being born in Birdie and Monica. Yet she still kept her eyes on her destiny to be a nurse.

Now we were ready to leave the apartment. I hugged Mary; and whispered in her ear, "I am so proud of you, and I love you very much." As we were walking out of the apartment, Monica raised her arms for me to pick her up and carry her to the car, and I did.

Birdie and Monica were too young to attend their mother's graduation ceremony. We dropped them off at mother's house on our way to the graduation ceremony at the St. Louis Kiel Auditorium, in downtown St. Louis, in the 1400 block of Clark Street.

My mom and dad were in the family room when we entered the house. Mother stood up and embraced Mary, giving her a lingering hug. She then stepped back, looked at Mary, and complimented her on how professional and attractive she looked in her nurse uniform. My niece Little Shirley agreed. My dad extended his congratulations and compliments as well.

Mary said, "Mother Drake, without everyone's help, I could not have achieved this goal." She sighed and said, "but God is good, and I know everything is possible through Him! That's the only way I, and we made it to this day."

I reminded Mary that it was getting late and she needed to be at the auditorium by 7:00 pm. Mother started laughing and said, "Mary, after all the effort you have gone through to finish school, I know you don't want to be one minute late for your graduation and getting your nurse's diploma."

Laughing, Mary said, "I know that's right, Mother Drake. Just think, me being blessed with these two little precious ones, who would have thought, I would finish nursing school." She quickly kissed the kids, and we left the house.

Driving to the Kiel Auditorium, we listened to the radio station KATZ. Mary was singing as the songs were playing and oozing with joy. Sitting next to her, I was basking in the thoughts of her accomplishment. We both were very upbeat and contemplating the graduation ceremony to conclude this long, challenging, but glorious journey of Mary becoming a Registered Nurse (RN).

When we arrived at the Kiel Auditorium, Mary was allowed to go in, but I had to wait until the doors were officially open to the general public at 7:00 pm. As the crowd grew larger, my decision to come early was prudent, and I was among the first to enter the auditorium when the doors were opened.

I found an aisle-row seat in the center section of the auditorium that was as close to the stage as possible. Mary's mother and her Aunt, Biddy, arrived later and were seated in a different area of the auditorium.

The graduation ceremony was a combined exercise with the nursing students from St. Louis City Hospital (#1) and Homer G. Phillips Hospital. A total of sixty-four students in the graduating class were from fourteen states in the United States (Missouri, Alabama, Illinois, Mississippi, Iowa, Texas, Ohio, Oklahoma, Tennessee, Michigan, Indiana, Arkansas, Kentucky, and Louisiana).

The Homer G. Director of Nursing, Miss. Minnie Edythe T. Gore presented the Homer G. Phillips nursing students with their graduation diplomas. When Mary's name was called, I knew her mother, and Aunt Biddy felt as proud of her, the same as I did.

147

To me, the expression of joy on Mary's face that Tuesday evening, September 22, 1964, was unforgettable, and her full persona was displayed. She strolled (sauntered) proudly across the Kiel Auditorium Opera House stage. Seemingly she was measuring each step, as they represented a true journey over the past five years of nursing school. With each step she took and her hand stretched out, she accepted her well-earned RN nursing diploma from Miss. Gore as part of the 1964 HGP class.

Mary persevered, and she was now graduating in the class of 1964. There were 31 student nurses that were in the 1964 HGP nursing school graduating class: Rita Allen, Josie M. Armstrong, Clara Barnes, Ikie H. Beamon, Freda L. Biggs, Herdesene Casher, Harvey N. Cline, Geraldine Cole, Mattie G. Davis, Ruth A. Dean, Mary A. Drake, Barrie J. English, Charlie F. Fisher, Annette Gray, Eva C. Hall, Joyce Y. Hart, Irsa Jackson, Dorothy M. Johnson, Jo Ann Lattier, Peggy J. Mason, Vivian May, Edna L. Moore, Patricia Sanderson, Beatrice M. Scott, Elizabeth Simms, Nancy Wilborne, Dorothy wills, Loretta Williams, Edna Jo Wilson, Jacqueline M. L. Wilson, Twana Young.

As I rejoiced in Mary's accomplishment, I detected a sense of pride on Miss. Gore's face. I wondered what thoughts were running through Miss. Gore's mind as she presented Mary with her well-earned graduation diploma. Was she thinking, "I knew you could do it, Miss. Byas-Drake." To a degree, I speculate that Mary finishing nursing school was, in effect, a personal accomplishment for Miss. Gore as well. Mary did not let her down.

Mary was now an "RN" among 26 or 27 nurses in her graduating class at HGP, which she was destined and determined to become. It was beyond her decision; I believe it was pre-determined. Mary only needed to complete her obligation to fulfill her spiritual destiny to become a nurse.

On graduation night, Mary and I did not have any celebration planned. Rather, Mary sort of sighed and gave a symbolic exhalation of gratefulness for the valiant road she (we) had traveled during the past five years.

Following her graduation ceremony, Mary immediately maneuvered through the crowd to come and hugged her mom and Aunt Biddy affectionately, thanking them for their support over the years. She kissed me and said, "I love you; thanks, babe!"

We left the auditorium and went to pick up the kids. When we entered the house, Monica was on the couch, half asleep. Birdie, with a big smile on his face asking "Momma, are you a nurse now?" Mary started laughing, kissed him, and said, " Yes, Birdie, I am a nurse!"

Then with a big smile on her face, she hugged mother and shared her emotional experience of walking across the stage to receive her nursing diploma. She showed off her RN Diploma. Little Shirley asked to see the Diploma, and Mary handed it to her. My dad was not a man that expressed many emotions; however, he was grinning as he congratulated Mary.

Mary tickled Monica and kissed her to wake her up completely. We said goodnight to my mom and dad and headed home. We arrived home late and put the kids to bed right away. Mary was still on an emotional high, and we talked for an hour or so, and we had an imaginary "champagne toast" to celebrate the occasion, and we went to bed.

The Missouri State Nursing Board Examination (MSNBE)

Now that school was over for Mary, I was thrilled to see her taking time to relax and unwind after her graduation. She was resting more, watching television late at night, and there was a drastic change in her routine. However, she knew that her leisure time would only last a couple of weeks, as she had to prepare to take the Missouri State Nursing Board Examination soon.

To become a certified RN, Mary had to pass the Missouri State Nursing Board Examination (MSNBE) after graduation. The state certification was required to be licensed as a "Registered Nurse" and to work in Missouri and other states in the United States.

The MSNBE is located in Jefferson City (JC), Missouri and Mary had to travel there to take the exam. Mary made hotel reservations at the Holiday

Inn Hotel. We planned to combine this trip with a long-deserved "mini extra-day vacation, to include celebrating Mary's graduation."

Mary and I both were looking forward to going to Jefferson City. This would be only our second trip together since we were married. Our first trip was to Memphis, Tennessee, in 1961 to introduce our son, Willis Drake Jr. (Birdie), who then was not yet a year old, to his great-grand-mother, Ma Dear (L. A. Sanford), so she could bless him.

That morning we dropped the kids off at mother's house and drove to Jefferson City. It was 135 miles, and the driving time would take us two hours and 40 minutes. We arrived and checked in at the hotel, and the accommodations were nice. There was a desk in the room, which made it convenient for Mary to review her exam notes in the evenings.

The Holiday Inn Hotel was within walking distance of the nursing board examination building, located at 3605 Missouri Blvd, Jefferson City, MO 65109, where Mary would take her exams. Several of Mary's class-mates were also taking the state exams, and they were staying at the same hotel where we stayed.

The Missouri State Nursing Board Examination (MSNBE) was a com-prehensive examination that would take three days to complete the five nursing disciplines of; Medical Nursing, Surgical Nursing, Obstetric Nursing, Nursing of Children, and Psychiatric Nursing. Mary had to extend her knowledge base back five years to cover the period when she first started her nursing training in 1959.

Not surprisingly, Mary passed the state nursing exams with scores well above the required standard scores. In fact, her scores for the psychiatric and Obstetric parts of the exam were "exceptionally high" compared to her other scores, which were also well above the state's average scores.

Following her third and final day of exams, Mary completed her state nurse's board examinations. Now with delight, we spent an extra day in Jefferson City to celebrate Mary's graduation.

We went out that evening and had dinner at a really lovely restaurant. The ambiance was mood-setting, the food was excellent, and we enjoyed the evening. When we returned to the hotel, we found a radio station that played R&B and Motown sounds, and the mood was set for a tremendous ending to conclude a fantastic enjoyable night!

CHAPTER 19

———— ◇ ————

Mary's First Registered Nurse (RN) Job

———— ◇ ————

FRESH FROM RETURNING HOME FROM Jefferson City, Mary would spend the next two weeks just relaxing and pampering Birdie and Monica. She was seriously contemplating getting a job soon. During this period, she received the exam results from her Missouri State Nursing Board Examination, exceeding the average score required on all five categories she was tested on.

Mary was now ready to start working and submitted applications for nursing positions at St. Louis City Visiting Nurses Program (SLCVNP) clinic, which was her preference, but there were no RN positions available. She also applied for a nursing position at DePaul Hospital.

DePaul is a Catholic hospital located at 2415 N. Kingshighway Boulevard at Highland Avenue. Its reputation as a medical institution within the community it serves was highly favorable. Tuesday evening, I came home from work, and Mary was elated, telling me, "Willis, I got a call this morning from DePaul Hospital asking me to come at 9:30 tomorrow morning for a job interview."

Her illuminating smile was captivating, and she said, "dinner is ready, babe, so let's eat while the food is hot, okay? I will tell you about my interview after we finish dinner." We had a wonderful meal, and after dinner, I played with the kids for a little while before Mary put them to bed.

Mary and I were relaxing on the couch in the living room, and I was stretch-out with my head resting in her lap. She was telling me the details of her telephone conversation with the DePaul Hospital representative. She sounded confident, stating, "I believe if I do well in my interview tomorrow, the hospital will offer me a nursing position." Hey, I will accept the job if I feel positive about the interview. I was neutral and said okay, that sounds good.

Mary had arranged for mother to watch the kids tomorrow morning. In the next breath, she said I have to get up early in the morning, get the kids dressed and take them to Mother Drake's. I could tell her mind was racing one hundred miles a minute. She was calm, and we then went to bed.

We rose early Wednesday morning, got dressed ourselves, and then got the kids up, and I helped get the kids dressed, and Mary fixed breakfast for them before I left for work. Mary would drop the kids at mother's house, and she would go for her job interview.

That evening when I got home from work, Mary was more reserved than usual. I immediately asked how the interview went, and she said, "Willis, it went okay. Then a smile caressed her face, and her exuberance was displayed. Baby, I aced the interview, and I was hired for the nursing position on the spot!" Then as if it was an afterthought, she kissed me as she usually did.

I responded and congratulated her, and asked, "How does it feel to have your first job as a Registered Nurse? When do you start working?" Hearing my voice, the kids converged in the living room, and I hugged them. Mary said, "okay, dinner is almost ready; let's wash up so we can eat, okay?

Mary told me and the kids at the dinner table that she would start her job next Monday. She emphasized to the kids that we would have a new daily routine now that she would be working. We will be getting up earlier in the mornings so that "your dad can take you to your grandmother's house before he goes to work. He will pick you up in the evenings like he did when I was in school, so be ready when he gets there, okay?

Smiling, Birdie said, "Monica, we can play with Wayne and little Shirley at grandmamma's house." With that stern look on her face, Mary said, "be obedient at your grandmother's house, and I know you will have fun playing with your cousins. Now that Mary had identified our new routine, we enjoyed a well-cooked dinner meal.

An incentive for Mary to work at DePaul initially was the convenience of her commute to work, which was a twenty-minute drive from our home. With Mary now working, it changed our family dynamics overall as well.

We shared in managing our daily household responsibilities. Before leaving for work in the mornings, Mary would put out food to cook for dinner that evening. Whoever got home first in the evening, and normally the kids and I did, would start cooking dinner.

When Mary got home from work that first day, the kids overwhelmed her when she walked into the house. Laughing playfully, she hugged and kissed them and told them to wash up so we could eat dinner. With laughter, I stated I worked hard my first day on the job and am hungry. "Willis, how much longer before we sit down to eat, babe? Everything is ready, so we can eat as soon as you wash up."

Monica no longer used her highchair and was sitting on the telephone books in her regular kitchen chair next to her mother. We enjoyed our meal while Mary explained how her first day at work went. Mostly, she had orientation in pediatrics and the OR (operating room) standard operating procedures processes. She also had instructions on the hospital's overall patient care operations.

The following months passed quickly, and Mary assimilated into her RN hospital duties very well over a year now. She worked mostly in the Operating Room (OR), which was not her preference. However, she performed her duties exceptionally well but did not enjoy working as an OR nurse.

She only said, "It was not pleasant for me to see a patient having surgery. She would laugh lightly and say, "Willis, that was a testament to me being trained at Homer G., one of the best nursing schools in the country, that I adjusted to all hospital situations very well."

The grapevine (network) among the RN fraternity, particularly among the Homer G. nurses alumni, was highly active. Mary was in the middle of her second year working at DePaul Hospital. Virginia (Vickie) Vaughn, Mary's former HGP classmate and close friend, worked as an RN in the North St. Louis City Visiting Nurse Program (VNP).

There were two St. Louis City VNP clinics; one was the North St. Louis City VNP, which serviced mostly the African American community, and the VPN clinic in South St. Louis, which serviced the predominately white community.

Vickie called Mary and told her that a VNP RN position was available where she worked at the Jefferson and Cass, North St. Louis City VNP clinic. Mary asked my thoughts if she should apply for the job, which she had coveted since graduating from nursing school. She was satisfied with her job at DePaul. However, she was confident she could help young girls that came to the VNP clinic for services.

Mary and I discussed and kicked around the pros and cons, and I was mostly a sounding board for her. She decided to apply for the VNP position. Mary had a job interview for the position and was hired. She talked with her Head Nurse first, and she gave DePaul Hospital her letter of resignation and two weeks' notice that she was resigning from her job. The hospital offered Mary a sizable pay increase to stay, but she declined their offer. She relished the opportunity of working with her close friend Vickie. They both were relatively new RNs with fresh ideas. They were willing to implement new and different nursing protocols, techniques, and thinking outside the rigid (box) lines.

Mary started her job at the North SLCVNP, and after one month, a trial program initiative was established within the SLCVNP clinic to educate teenage girls regarding pregnancy prevention. A medical doctor outside the SLCVNP was hired to head-up the new trial program.

The doctor recruited from the SLCVNP for two registered nurses to operate the trial program. The nurses would set up and implement the policies, concepts, and procedures established by the doctor and the medical administration.

Vickie and Mary discussed and collaborated on the merits of working in the new "pregnancy prevention type program" and the benefit it could provide to the teenage community, particularly African-American teenagers. They agreed to transfer to the new program. The senior and experienced nurses at the SLCVNP supported their decision.

With lofty expectations, Vickie and Mary had their initial meeting with the doctor heading up the program. He identified the program's objectives and what he expected from the two RNs overseeing the program's daily operation. He emphasized the program's purpose and supported their discretion in providing recommended informational material to teenage clients referred by the Visiting Nurse Program.

The doctor usually came to the clinic twice a week and would conduct an hour-long staff meeting with Vickie and Mary. In lieu of providing them with specific guidance and policy information they needed, he would obfuscate, telling them to use their professional judgment to perform their jobs.

As the trial program got off the ground, Vickie and Mary coordinated and organized their individual offices and collaborated with the VNP nurses and clinical staff. They wanted to create synergy between the two programs. Vickie and Mary worked extremely well together and received positive acknowledgment from the VNP clinical staff for the trial program.

They provided educational information to answer the young teenagers' questions and debunked misinformation based on total ignorance.

Vickie and Mary would also help educate young mothers on how to properly care for their new babies and provide needed resource information. They also established an excellent rapport with the teenagers receiving services at the SLCVNP.

Mary Was Unjustly Fired From Her Job

Everything was on point in our lives! We had a happy marriage with two normal healthy, developing young children, a supportive family, and close personal friends, and we were satisfied with our professional careers.

Mary had been working for several months at her new job. On this particular Friday evening, she came home from work, and things were "turned upside down." Mary walked into the apartment as she normally did; however, she was not smiling and looked despondent! The event that day on her job had changed drastically for her.

She just stood in the doorway for a minute and was slow to close the door behind her. She did not greet me or the kids in her usual happy demeanor. She reacted solemnly, like a person in a mental fog and distraught. The events of that evening are still vivid in my memory.

Willis Jr. always allowed Monica to hug their mother first when she got home. Mary's reaction to their greeting was different this evening. She did not display that radiant, happy welcome in seeing her babies. Then in the next breath, she said, "momma is a little tired. Can you go to your room and play? I will come to see you in a few minutes, okay?"

I approached to kiss her, and she manufactured a forced smile. Looking into her eyes revealed that something was seriously wrong. I never got to embrace her with a hug, as usual. She said softly, "Willis, I was fired from my job today!"

I embraced her gently and guided her to the couch to sit down. Her countenance was flushed, and I could see the pain in her face as I held her hand. "Are you all right? What happened, baby? I inquired.

Sitting down, Mary was slightly composed now. She stated, "Willis, the doctor came into the clinic this afternoon and immediately summoned me to his office. I went into his office with an upbeat frame of mind. However, as soon as I sat down in the chair, he said, 'Mrs. Drake, I am going to let you go. Today is your last day, and I need you to leave anything that belongs to the clinic in your office.'

"Willis, I had an ill feeling come over me. The way the doctor so matter-of-factly informed me that he was firing me without giving me an explanation was appalling. I had a horrible feeling in the pit of my stomach sitting in his office and felt like I was going to throw up."

She stated emphatically, "Willis, there isn't a valid reason I was fired. I have not done anything to justify being fired." Mary's eyes were now moist with tears, and she said, "Willis, I asked the doctor what I had done wrong to be fired?" He said, "I don't want to discuss it further. I made the decision, and you are terminated effective immediately."

"Baby, I stood up with poise and my head high as I walked out of his office and stayed calm. I felt like crying, but I fought back the tears. I would not let that doctor see one tear fall from my eyes. I would not give him the satisfaction of knowing that his fraudulent termination action against me had penetrated my emotional barrier.

Willis, I know I was doing a terrific service for the young teenagers I worked with. I love my job, and I know I was making a positive difference in the lives of the teenagers I came in contact with daily.

When I came from the doctor's office, I immediately told Vickie what had just happened. She was upset and was going to quit her job right there on the spot. I persuaded her not to react irrationally over what had happened to me. I told her, "I will go home and talk with you, and I know everything will be all right."

Listening to Mary, I was contemplating how to handle this situation, to rectify this injustice. Knowing Mary, it was absolutely inconceivable that she had done anything to be fired. It was unfair for her to be fired for no valid reason. I firmly believe that the arc of justice bends mightily in favor of right! Therefore, I knew "right" would prevail from this doctor's imperious action against Mary.

As we talked, Mary obviously was feeling better having our conversation. She rose from the couch, and her voice was now normal. She called out, where are my two little munchkins, as she went to their bedroom, saying, "where are you? Where are you? As she reached their bedroom. I see you; there you are." She hugged Monica and Birdie, kissing them repeatedly.

With the kids wrapped in her arms, she said, "I am hungry. Are you guys hungry too?" Tickling Monica's stomach, she said let's wash up so we can eat dinner. We ate dinner, and Mary had her playtime with the kids after we finished eating. A little while later, she put Birdie and Monica to bed.

I was only one year older than Mary, but she always believed that I could fix any wrong that happened to us. Mary and I went to the living room to discuss the ramifications of her being fired; and what recourse she had. Mary was at ease as we sat on the living room couch talking. We both were calm, discussing the options we had to address the situation. Finally, after kicking around what we thought, I told Mary that I would call my mother's attorney; Arthur (Art) Friedman, to get his legal advice regarding what recourse was available to Mary.

Mary repeated over and over, "Willis, I have searched my mind deeply, to think of anything that I had done to warrant being fired. However, there is absolutely nothing that I can think of that would justify my losing my job!"

It is conceivable that Mary's pleasant personality, and cooperating attitude, may be misconstrued and misinterpreted by certain individuals, who may want to elevate themselves at her expense. Possibly people in general, and that mendacious doctor in particular, misunderstood, or miscalculated, that Mary would not stand up for herself; and demand justice for an unfair termination action against her.

However, more than anything, the doctor did not understand that Mary's husband was not as hospitable if anyone mistreated Mary. My philosophy and theory have always been that when you are in the right, you will prevail over wrongdoings. In my eyesight, that "doctor" was inconsequential, and he had inappropriately fired Mary and had encroached on her "life's dream."

I became incensed thinking that this doctor, on a claptrap whim, thought he could exert unfair action against Mary with impunity. He obliviously had no idea that Mary Ann Byas-Drake had endured five years to complete her RN training. Plus, during that time, she had become a mother twice, and still, she was able to finish nursing school and become a registered nurse! Additionally, that doctor did not understand that something much bigger than him, a "Spiritual element," was part of Mary's life's journey. She was "destined and determined" to be a nurse!

Early Saturday morning, Mary, the kids, and I drove to my parent's home. After our good morning acknowledgements, in short order, mother, Mary, and I went to the kitchen to talk, and my dad was in the family room watching Birdie and Monica.

Sitting at the kitchen table, Mary, with tears in her eyes, said, "Mother Drake, I was fired from my job yesterday." Observing the expression on mother's face, she was astonished. In a serious and bewildered voice, she asked, "Mary, what happened? Why were you fired?"

Wiping her eyes, Mary responded, "Mother Drake, that's what's so aggravating. The doctor, my supervisor, did not give me a reason why he fired me. He came to the clinic yesterday and called me into his office, and told me I was fried effective immediately. I asked why I was being fried, but he would not give me any justification for his action."

With more composure now, Mary assured mother "that she hasn't done anything to justify being terminated from her job." Mother was really hot (upset). She said, "that doctor must be a fool!" I told mother we wanted to contact your attorney Arthur (Art) Friedman, to seek legal advice. Can you give me his telephone number, please?

She got her telephone book and gave me Art's phone number. Be sure to let Art know that you are my son, and Mary is my daughter-in-law. We returned to the family room, and my dad had a concerned look on his face. He asked if everything was okay. Mother said, "Yes, Kermit, I will talk with you later." Mary and I got the kids and left the house to go home.

We arrived back at the apartment, and with the kids' activity levels elevated, we took them to the park to burn off their energy. An hour later, we returned home and spent our weekend as normally as possible. Later that evening, Mary and I discussed contacting attorney Art Friedman Monday morning.

It had been an emotional meandering weekend. Our Monday morning routine was altered slightly as I dropped Willis Jr. at mother's house so he could attend school. Mary kept Monica home with her. At work around 10:00 am, I called Attorney Arthur (Art) Friedman's office. I told his secretary I was Mrs. Kermit Drake's son and asked to speak to Attorney Art Friedman.

A few minutes later, Art was on the phone asking, "how can I help you?" I told him, "I want to schedule an appointment for my wife, Mary Byas-Drake; she needs your legal advice regarding a wrongful termination from her job."

Art asked where my wife worked. I explained that "Mary is a registered nurse, and she was working for the St. Louis City Visiting Nurse Program (SLCVNP). However, last Friday, she was fired from her job. We need your advice regarding her options to correct this unjustified termination action taken against her."

He responded quickly, "Okay, Mr. Drake, have your wife come to my office tomorrow at 10:00 am. I will need her to provide the details of what happened regarding her job termination. Tell your mother hello." I thanked Attorney Friedman and hung up the phone.

I immediately called Mary to let her know that she had an appointment to meet with Art Friedman tomorrow morning at ten o'clock. She sounded enthused, and we decided to talk in more detail when I got home this evening.

After work, I picked up Willis Jr. from mother's house and headed home. Arriving home, Mary was anxious to discuss her meeting tomorrow with attorney Friedman. I had to slow her down, so we would first have dinner as usual. After everything had quieted down and the kids went to bed, we would discuss Mary's meeting with Art tomorrow.

Mary and I later discussed the details she needed to inform Art Friedman regarding her job termination. Mary made copious notes to discuss with attorney Friedman during their meeting. I gave Mary directions to Art's law firm office in downtown St. Louis, in the 1100 block of Pine Street.

I asked Mary if she wanted me to accompany her to meet with the Attorney. I could take off work for a couple of hours in the morning. Mary assured me that she would be fine meeting with Art alone. "Willis, since I will be downtown near your workplace tomorrow after the meeting, can I stop at your job and let you know how the meeting went?" Yes, that will be great, baby.

On Tuesday morning, I got ready for work, and Mary also got up and got dressed herself. She also had to get the kids ready to take them to mother's house.

As I was leaving the house, I wished Mary good luck with her meeting with Art. I let her know that I would see her around eleven o'clock after she finished her meeting.

Mary came to my workplace as planned after her meeting was over. This was the first time she had ever come to my job. She walked casually from

MARY'S FIRST REGISTERED NURSE (RN) JOB

the elevator to my desk, elegantly dressed, and looked very professional and attractive as always.

She sat in my guest chair, and as she observed my work area, she commented that she knew several of my coworkers who lived in East St. Louis and went to high school with her.

Mary then immediately turned her attention to her meeting with attorney Friedman. She was smiling unabashedly as she recounted, "Attorney Friedman's secretary escorted me into his interoffice. Willis, I was flabbergasted when I saw Attorney Art Friedman!

Do you remember in my senior year of nursing school, I had to spend three weeks at the South St. Louis nurse's campus? Part of the course curriculum was I had to sit in on court cases at the St. Louis City Courts as part of my nurses' training.

Willis, do you recall me telling you about this one case where the defense attorney picked apart the prosecutor's case against his client so skillfully? I was so impressed with that defense attorney.

Willis, can you imagine when I walk into Art Friedman's office and I am face-to-face with this same defense attorney; I had extolled as this brilliant Lawyer; I had observed in court during my senior year of nursing school. Willis, Art sat across the conference table from me with a legal pad in front of him. As he introduced himself, he said, 'you are Mrs. Drake's daughter-in-law, right?'

Then he asked me, 'what happened, and why were you terminated?' Willis, I reiterated verbatim, describing to attorney Friedman what the doctor (my supervisor) said when he fired me. I also emphasized that the doctor refused to discuss or give me a reason why he was terminating me. At this point, attorney Art Friedman now had a smile on his face and said, 'I am certain, based on what you have described, Mrs. Drake, your termination will be corrected.'

Willis, I had never considered it, but Art asked me if I wanted to file a lawsuit against the city for a monetary settlement. Without hesitating, I told him, "no," I am not interested in suing the city. I just want my job back as a registered nurse, and I want my record cleared up regarding my termination. Also, I don't want to work in the office with that doctor.

Willis, we finished our meeting in 30 minutes, and I thanked attorney Friedman for taking my case. As I was leaving, he walked me to his office door and said, 'when my investigator completes his work, I will update you on the status of your case early next week.'"

Mary had been at my job for 15 minutes when she said, "I have to pick up Monica from Mother Drake's. Willis, I will see you when you get home this evening. I walked her to the elevator, and I knew that justice would be rendered correctly on her behalf. I knew that "truth" would prevail in Mary's situation.

Mary was enjoying her time at home with Monica. Less than two weeks later, attorney Art Friedman called and informed Mary that he had a meeting with the appropriate St. Louis City legal representatives, and her case had been settled, and her termination had been reversed totally without any complications.

Art Friedman told Mary, "Your case against the doctor was "indisputable" and that's why it was settled so quickly. The doctor didn't have any legitimate justification for terminating you. There was no logical and most certainly no legal explanation for his erroneous action against you. He was exposed for his fraudulent action. Mrs. Drake, the city was fortunate that you didn't want to file a lawsuit against them for monetary damages.

Just to let you know, Mrs. Drake, my legal investigator spoke with "the professional medical staff, administrators, and the clerical support staff at the clinic. In every instance, they had the highest exemplary comments about you."

As you demanded, you are immediately restored to your visiting nurse job. You will not be working in the office with that doctor. A position at the South St. Louis Public Health Visiting Nurse Program (SLPHVNP) has been made available for you. Plus, your personnel records will not reflect any reference to the erroneous termination action taken against you. The record of that tainted action has been expunged permanently from your personnel file," he concluded.

Mary thanked attorney Friedman, and the favorable resolution of her case restored Mary's enthusiasm for working again with young teenagers. Being assigned to the South St. Louis SLPHVNP clinic, I believe she was possibly the first or one of the first African-American RN public health visiting nurses to work at that clinic.

Mary had to drive 25 minutes longer to get to her job at the South St. Louis clinic; than she did working at the Jefferson and Cass clinic. Her commuting distance in miles, driving to South St. Louis, also increased by twice the miles she previously had to drive to work.

In a reasonably short time, Mary connected professionally with many of the young teenage girls registered at the clinic. This was regardless of their ethnicity and racial background. As she built up their trust, she gained their confidence as well. Age-wise at twenty-six years old, Mary was positioned perhaps strategically better than the other older nurses working in the clinic. Likely, her firsthand experience as a teenage wife and mother was germane in performing her job effectively.

So, working in South St. Louis, Mary professionally planted her feet on solid ground. However, she quickly established herself in a favorable position on the job with her clients, staff members, and coworkers.

As she got to know the clinic's clients, Mary now had firsthand knowl-edge of what she already knew. The existence of teenage pregnancy among a population of white teenage girls' was also prevalent in this south St. Louis community. This was similar to what was the situation in the African-American Jefferson-Cass community. It was an overall common teenage problem concern.

Ostensibly Mary was recognized among her peers as a knowledgeable, dedicated nurse and team member. Arriving home each day, she had a story of success that had motivated her professionally at work and satisfied her personally on the job.

Time passed, and Mary continued being a dedicated nurse, doing her job at the South St. Louis clinic. She received personal satisfaction as she continued to inspire young teenage mothers to move forward with their lives productively and positively.

Mary had compassion for helping young teenagers, as she advised and encouraged them to eradicate any negative behavior in their lives. She demonstrated, through various means, how young teenagers could reach their potential in life after experiencing a "mistake."

It was good to see that Mary's job was gratifying for her, day in and day out, and she was blessed to be a nurse!

The Doctor Fired
Mary's awful experience at her last job was only several weeks removed from the present time. With her new position at the South St. Louis clinic and our focus on buying our first house, the ramification of her former job was a thing of the past. She had totally put that situation behind her now.

Mary had been working at the South St. Louis clinic for less than two months. This particular evening when she came home from work, she had a devilish smile on her face. She said, "Vickie (Virginia "Vickie" Vaughn), her best friend and her former co-worker called me today and told me that her supervisor, "the doctor," was fired today.

I asked what had happened. Why did he get fired?" Mary, with a look of redemption on her face, said I don't know. Vickie doesn't have the details yet, but she will tell me more later, I am sure. Mary said, "devious and dishonest people with ill intentions towards others will reap what they sow. The consequence of their actions often ends with something negative happening to them."

Amazingly after Mary was assigned to her South St. Louis clinic job, the subject of "that doctor's" fiasco was not discussed in our household. I am sure that Vickie and Mary discussed why that doctor was fired at some point. It's amazing how Mary was quickly "vindicated" from an underhanded action, and shortly thereafter, the perpetrator of that unjust action, the doctor himself, was fired.

CHAPTER 20

$\diamondsuit$

Our Social Life

$\diamondsuit$

M ARY HAD ENDURED THE EXTREME rigor of nursing school for five years. Now she was a working mom, and the kids were approaching kindergartner and elementary school age. As a young married couple, we relished "having fun and enjoying life with our kids and family members."

We were not heavy partygoers and were not real "drinkers." I would have a beer or a cocktail at a party. Mary didn't drink alcoholic beverages; however, she would enjoy a "Virgin (non-alcohol) Strawberry Daiquiri" at parties.

As a young (ages 24 & 25) energetic couple, we relished having a "night out" to enjoy ourselves. Our social buddies were Mary's closest friends and former nursing school classmates; Virginia (Ruth), Vickers-Vaughn (Vickie), and Florence (Jean) Charleston-Washington were also married and had a young child. We as a group would have an evening out periodically to socialize and have fun.

I had a close friendship with their husbands, Marvin Vaughn, and Ronald (Ronnie) Washington. They both were cool dudes, good husbands, and fathers. Our families had similar interests and shared a solid social relationship. My lifelong friend, Stanley McKissic, and his wife, Gladys, were always included in our social gatherings also.

Generally, we were the same age and came from similar social, educational, and economic backgrounds and lifestyles. Each couple had a young child between the ages of two and six.

Marvin and Vickie's daughter, Vivian, "little Vickie," was the oldest among the kids. Willis Jr. was a few years younger; Ronnie and Jean's daughter, Angela (Angie), was months younger than Willis Jr.; our daughter Monica was a year younger than Angie. Marvin Vaughn Jr. was not born yet.

Twice a month, we alternated weekends, rotating from one couple's home to the next couple's home. Many African-Americans in our generation played the card game "Bid-Whist," which was broadly played on HBCU (Historically Black Colleges and Universities) campuses, nursing school dormitories, and individuals' homes.

On Friday evenings, usually at seven o'clock, we would get together at the host's home to play Bid-Whist. Our kids enjoyed playing with one another and were part of our fun Friday weekend activity.

The host couple provided food, beverages, and entertainment (radio music or records) for the gathering. We normally had open-face sandwiches, party snacks, and the like. As a group, we were not hard liquor drinkers, and we had beer and soft drinks available. Playing "Bid-Whist" was the primary entertainment. When the parents were not playing a "hand of cards" at the time, each parent shared equally in keeping an eye watching all the children.

The fun of bid-whist was "instigating, talking smack and signifying during the card game." Ronnie and I would play together as partners, and when we had a "roadmap" hand, we would show out and clown. Our evening of fun and entertainment was upbeat, laughing and kidding around, plus it was an inexpensive evening. Usually, we ended the evening around 11:00–11:30 pm.

Mary was always arranging with our friends Vickie and Jean to take our children bowling, roller-skating, and to the St. Louis zoo and on picnics at Forest Park and other public parks in St. Louis.

CHAPTER 21

--- ◇ ---

Lake of the Ozarks—Vacation

--- ◇ ---

B Y NECESSITY, MORE SO THAN by design, Mary and I had foregone personal vacation time that young married couples often would enjoy during the first six years of our marriage. Having two children during the time Mary started and graduated nursing school, taking a vacation was not an option.

As young adults in our early twenties, Mary and I enjoyed having fun like most young couples. However, we were not "partygoers" and didn't routinely frequent nightclubs and lounges for our entertainment. Mary's brother David (Byas) periodically babysat Birdie and Monica so we could have an evening out.

With Mary and I employed, we were now economically considered middle-class. We had the discretionary financial resources available to enjoy certain entertainment activities, including taking a week's summer vacation annually.

During the sixties (1960s), there were limited public outlets or facilities for professional and middle-class African-American individuals or families to socialize. There were several prominent African-American social clubs in St. Louis, and they owned property where they held their club meetings and other social activities they sponsored.

There was limited access that African-Americans had to recreational facilities in general, specifically that was located in the Lake of the Ozarks area. Mr. Frank Gibson, an African-American civil service employee, worked at the Mart Building, where I also worked. He was the secretary-treasurer of his social club.

Mr. Gibson's social club built and owned a lakefront "cabin" in the Lake of the Ozarks area. The use of their cabin was primarily for their club member's benefit. However, they would rent the cabin to responsible individuals for a very reasonable rental fee.

At the beginning of the year (1967), Mary wanted us to take a vacation in June without the kids. She put in a request for her vacation time for June, and I submitted my request on my job, and our vacations were approved. Now the spring of the year was on the cusp of rolling into the summer. I was bent on giving Mary a well-deserved summer vacation in June. This would be our first vacation without having our children with us.

Some of my white coworkers, and casual friends, often described their weekend at the Lake of the Ozarks. They talked about their fabulous time at the Ozarks with their wives, walking on the beach and swimming in the lake. Hearing my coworkers talk about the fun they had at the Lake of the Ozarks, I thought it would also be a terrific place for our vacation.

I talked to Mr. Gibson in mid-May about renting his social club's cabin in the Lake of the Ozarks. When I walked into his office, he had that engaging smile and said, as usual, "hello, young fellow." That was the moniker of respect that he had for me. We laughed and chatted for a few minutes, and I asked if I could rent his club's cabin for the week of June 18th.

Mr. Gibson talked about the racial overtones and the antics the local community initially engaged in to prevent their social club from purchasing the "beachfront property" on the lake. He said, "Despite the attempts, our club was able to purchase the land and build our cabin

172

from the ground up. It is one of the best-looking cabins in that area at the Lake of the Ozarks."

Willis, the club, normally doesn't rent the cabin to young people. We are particular about our club's image because the local community would focus on anything negative happening at our property. However, Willis, I know you and your guests will socialize and enjoy yourselves the same as our club members would. Yes, I will rent the cabin to you."

I wanted to surprise Mary with the news when I got home. At the dinner table, I told Mary I had rented a "cabin" at the Lake of the Ozarks for our vacation in June. She was ecstatic, and then Monica shouted, "momma Birdie and I want to go too." Mary chuckled, pinched Monica's little cheek, and said politely, "baby girl, this vacation is just for your dad and me, okay?"

Mary and I would vacation together with my sister Shirley and her husband Stanley (Stan) Sykes and our friends Vickie and Marvin (Vaughn). Mary called Shirley and Vickie to let them know our vacation reservation at the Lake of the Ozarks was confirmed. I heard the laughing and chatter while Mary was talking on the phone. Apparently, Shirley and Vicki were as excited as Mary was.

Later that evening, Mary went to her closet and got this "yellow swimsuit" and said, "it's your favorite color for me. Willis, I know I can't swim a lick, but I bought this swimsuit to wear on the beach at the Lake of the Ozarks. What do you think, babe? I hope you will like how I look in it."

I smiled and said, "I can imagine just how "fine" you will look in that yellow swimsuit, girl! To me, you look fine in anything yellow that you wear. Maybe I can teach you to swim while we're on vacation. Mary laughed and said that would be a miracle.

Finally, Monday, June 18th, was here. We had to drive roughly 175 miles to the cabin, and it would take us about three hours to get there. The six of us would ride together in my car.

The radio was on as we drove to the cabin, and the music kept us entertained most of the way. As we got closer to our destination, we turned off the radio, and we were focused on the directions to the cabin. Mr. Gibson had given excellent directions, and we had a safe trip driving to the cabin.

After a comfortable but long drive, we arrived at the cabin, got out of the car, and stressed our legs. The women went in and walked through, inspecting every inch of the cabin. After a few minutes, there was a collective resounding "wow" this cabin looks terrific.

The cabin had three bedrooms, a large modern kitchen, and a spacious living room with a TV and radio, with top-quality furniture throughout the cabin. The ladies, individually, selected the bedroom where each of us would sleep. Mary and I got the "Master Bedroom."

After we got situated in the cabin, we drove to the local grocery store to purchase food for our week's stay. We were now self-sufficient to enjoy the week at the Lake of the Ozarks.

That first evening, Mary and I took a walk on the beach wearing the casual clothes we had traveled in; and observing the surrounding areas where we were staying. We were the only African-Americans on the Lake of the Ozarks that day. I noticed day after day, as we went down to the beach, we were still the only African-Americans in the area.

We had exceptional lodging accommodations, and we relaxed in comfort, in or out of the cabin. However, we went to the beach every day. I felt proud, seeing Mary in her yellow swimsuit, and looking great. She was splashing in the water, no deeper than to her knees. She was laughing and having fun pretending she was swimming. It was the same with Shirley and Vickie, looking great in their swimsuits, but couldn't swim. Stan, Marvin, and I were feasting our eyes on our wives.

We were having a terrific vacation as the week was wounding down. We had retired for the night, and Mary said, "Baby, I will never forget that vacation. It will always be etched in my memory like indelible ink." We laughed, and I said, "Babe, although we have been married six years, this trip is really like our honeymoon that we never had." Mary agreed as we cuddled and went to sleep.

That Thursday and Friday, many more people were on the beach, and people were just having fun. Also, we saw another African American, and even more astonishing, it was Richard Shelton. Richard and I attended Lane Tabernacle CME Church as kids, and we were in the same Sunday school class together.

Richard was spending the weekend in a cabin with friends near the cabin where we were staying. So I knew other African-Americans were there for the weekend.

However, what I remember most about that entire weekend was standing in the Lake of the Ozarks, with water up to my knees. Mary was wearing her "yellow swimsuit," and I was holding her in my arms, and my muscles were bulging. She was looking so fine with her sunglasses on, and her beautiful smile caressed her face. Now that is the image that is etched on my brain that I will always remember.

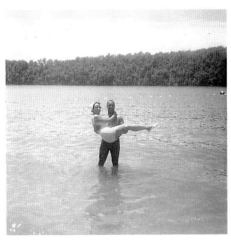

Lake of the Ozarks (Willis holding Mary)

CHAPTER 22

◇

Buying Our First Home

◇

F ROM 1964 TO 1969, MARY'S professional nursing career allowed
her to work as an Operating Room (OR), Special Programs Nurse,
and a St. Louis City Public Health (Visiting) Nurse. She was en-
thralled with her nursing career, which allowed her to help people. Additionally, she was committed to and subscribed to the plan, goal, and
vision I had for our family to purchase our first home.

We had decided early in our marriage to save money to purchase our
house in the near future. Mary had been very patient in following our
saving plan and waiting until our "money was right" before we started
looking to buy a house. Along the way, now and then, Mary was tempt-
ed, wanting to look to buy a house sooner than our plan indicated.

However, with a little persuasion, I was always able to convince her to
stay the course of purchasing our house. However, we both appreciated
having "nice" possessions and material things now for our family to
enjoy our good fortunes and blessings.

Since I was eight years old, I would work and save my nickels and
dimes to pay for anything I wanted to buy for myself. This habit, or ingrained practice, continued with me as a teenager. This concept, plan,
or approach was part of my emblematic fabric. When Mary was in

nursing school, we would save the money first, to purchase anything we wanted.

Mary, through assimilation, adapted to my concept. Now we both ascribed to this save first and buy later approach in purchasing what we needed to acquire.

In 1967, I suffered a reduction in my annual income. Our roles were reversed financially, and Mary's annual income was greater than mine. Therefore, we recalculated our financial situation; and started saving my income; and we began living from Mary's income for our daily, monthly, and annual subsistence needs.

Routinely as husband and wife, Mary and I worked together in everything. There was no "yours and mine" scenario. We had the same single-mindedness in planning to buy our first house, as well as saving for our children's college education. With this change in my income status, it would take maybe a few years longer to buy our house than we had previously projected.

There was no lingering "ego trip" with me because Mary's income was now higher than mine. However, what I have always known, from a spiritual aspect, I knew this to be true because I had witnessed it first-hand. When untoward things happened to me, as was the case in my salary reduction, it would be rectified.

A year later, in 1968, I got a job at the Army Mobility Equipment Command (MECOM), and my salary (possibly unprecedented) increased by four grade levels. Now my annual salary was more than Mary's salary. However, we continued living on Mary's income to support our family household needs; and continued saving my annual income. Therefore, we could start looking to buy our first house sooner than we had initially planned.

Financially, there was fluidity in our weekly budget. With dedicated financial planning over the years, we had the luxury of providing more discretionary funds for our kids, possibly more than our contemporaries could provide for their children. Mary was not an extravagant person, and I was fugal regarding our normal spending. So we had the disposable income available, which did not impact our weekly budget outlays or savings.

When we decided to buy our house, no real estate agency was initially involved in assisting us in finding a house. So we used the Sunday weekend newspapers to find houses listed for sale in the geographical areas where we were interested in living. We decided north St. Louis County was where we would focus our attention on buying a house.

At the time, St. Louis real estate agencies seemed to steer African-American families to University City to purchase houses. We, however, decided to look for a house in the North-West County, St. Louis metropolitan area that included Florissant, Missouri, approximately forty-five minutes from downtown St. Louis.

In 1969 there were only a few African-American families living in the Florissant area. As first-time prospective home buyers, our fundamental process was to drive through a community where we were interested in buying a house. Then if we saw a house listed for sale and we wanted to see the inside, we would contact the real estate agency and schedule an appointment.

In the late 1960s (1968 or 1969), St. Louis local newspapers reported racial incidents where an African-American family bought a home in the suburban white community in Jennings, MO. The day the African-American family moved into their house, white racists burned a cross on the front lawn of their home.

Mary and I first looked at houses in Berkeley and Ferguson, Missouri. Reflecting now, I think, "wow," we had considered buying a home on St. Elizabeth Street in Ferguson, MO. This was in 1969, forty-plus years before the 2014 racial incident in Ferguson, MO.

We only seriously considered two houses before we bought the house located at 1340 Mullanphy Lane in Florissant, MO. Routinely Mary and I always looked at houses together. However, I saw a house for sale listed in a local St. Louis county newspaper. Normally I would discuss with Mary the house's location and any other pertinent information before contacting the realtor.

It was a Friday evening around 5:00 pm, and I had just gotten off work. I am not certain what prompted me to call the realtor's office, but I did. The real estate agent answered the phone, and I told him I was interested in seeing the house listed for sale on Mullanphy Lane.

With a slight pause in responding, he said, "It's late, and I am in the office alone. If you can get here by 6:30 pm, I will stay and show you the house." I do not recall the name of the real estate agency. The agent gave me excellent directions to his Dunn and Pershall Road office.

It was the evening rush hour. The highway was crowded, and I was unfamiliar with this area of highway I-70 west. My directions to the real estate office were precise, and I pulled into the parking lot at 6:15 pm.

I entered the realtor's office, and the agent was leaning back in his desk chair with his right foot on his desk. He was facing the window and reading a newspaper. He looked up, and the expression on his face when he saw me indicated he was surprised that I was an African-American.

Standing in front of his desk, I introduced myself. "My name is Willis Drake, and we spoke on the phone regarding the house on Mullanphy Lane." He politely introduced himself, and we shook hands. He was a tall, slender built man in his early fifties with mingled gray hair.

He was cordial and asked if I was familiar with the Florissant area. "That traffic was horrible at this time of evening, and the house was fifteen minutes away. Mr. Drake, you can ride in my car to go see the house."

Driving to the house, the agent chatted politely about the nice neighborhood, and there was a school within walking distance of the house located at 1340 Mullanphy Lane. The major thoroughfare near the house was Lindbergh Boulevard. As I listened to the agent, I was checking out the community in general and the overall neighborhood environment as we were driving.

The agent and I did not talk much; however, I recall him saying, "When you see the house, and if you are interested in buying the house. I would want you to put a deposit on the house, to keep another agent from showing the house to someone else." I never responded with a comment.

He pulled into the driveway. I do not know why, but I had a special feeling about the house before I got out of the car. The house from the outside immediately appealed to me. It was a red brick ranch-style house with an attached one-car garage, a well-kept front lawn, with a big tree in the front yard.

The agent opened the front door, and I had not yet crossed the threshold. Just looking into the house from the doorway, I was instantly impressed with the house. It was as if I had been guided to this house intentionally, and I knew it was the house for us to buy.

On the upper level of the house, there were three bedrooms, a living room, an informal dining room, a kitchen, a full bathroom off the main hallway, and the master bedroom had a half bathroom. There was a regular size kitchen with an archway that separated the semi-formal dining room from the kitchen.

There was a large full basement; half of the basement had been finished with a tiled floor, wood-paneled walls, and an acoustic ceiling. There was a large enough fenced backyard with a privacy fence on the left side of the patio. The back and front lawns were well-kept.

I probably walked through the house in fifteen minutes, and I had the feeling that this was "the house we would buy." I was hoping when Mary saw the house; she would have the same feelings about it as I do.

We were driving back to his office, and the agent was more talkative. He asked if I liked the house and if I was interested in buying it. I was casual with my response and told him the house has some features we were looking for. I want to bring my wife to see the house, and then we will let him know if we are interested in buying it.

I asked for a blank copy of the contract he wanted me to sign. He looked puzzled and asked why I needed a blank contract, which was not normally done. I stated, "my attorney needs to look over the contract before I commit to purchasing the house. That I wanted to have the house inspected, at my expense, to ensure, construction-wise, that the house was sound. I wanted to be certain there were no hidden problems with the house. Reluctantly, the realtor gave me a blank copy of the contract.

Arriving home, I was excited to tell Mary about this house, and I wanted her to see it as soon as possible. Mary was always enthused about going to see houses, regardless if she was interested in buying the house or not.

After describing the house to Mary, I called the realtor and scheduled an appointment for Mary and me to look at the house. The traffic was not as congested that Saturday morning when we went to see the house. I recall initially that Mary liked the house, but she was not as enthused and blown away by it, the same as I was.

After seeing the house, Mary and I seriously discussed if we wanted to buy the house. We decided to go back and look at the house a third time, and we took Willis Jr. and Monica with us, so they could see the house.

This time we meticulously went through the house. Mary took room measurements and window sizes and speculated where the furniture would be placed in each room. I could tell that she wanted this house the same as I did.

With her created imagination, Mary started to visualize and articulate verbally how she would decorate the house. She would make a rhetorical comment and then solicit my opinion but not expect a reply from me. Monica was by her mother's side supporting every idea Mary espoused. Willis Jr. and I were basically silent on the furniture and how the house would be decorated.

Mary and I agreed we would make an offer to buy the house located at "1340 Mullanphy Lane, Florissant, Mo." However, the one thing Mary wanted was new carpet in the living room and dining room prior to moving into the house.

I contacted our Attorney, Arthur Friedman (Art), to look over the blank real estate contract. He advised that the blank real estate contract was standard. If we wanted to buy the house, signing the contract would be no problem.

Art also had his construction investigator, who was also a home construction (builder) developer contractor, inspect the house. He did a detailed inspection of the house, and his report documented that construction and foundation-wise, the house was in excellent condition.

Art also stated that his investigator said, "We were getting a remarkable deal on the price of the house." It turned out that Art's construction investigator personally knew the house's owner. He was also a home construction developer contractor. He (now owned the house) had taken the house as a trade-in on a new house that he had built and sold to the former owner of the house at 1340 Mullanphy Lane.

It was also interesting that the person that previously owned the house was James (Jim) Pender. Jim and I had worked together at the Mart Building a few years ago during the early 1960s when we both worked for the Daily Record Company on the GSA contract. Charles (Charlie) Moore, James (Jim) Heffington, and James (Jim) Pender were good friends from high school at that time.

On this occasion, as was the case whenever we made a major decision. Mary and I went to my parent's home to let them know that we had found the house we wanted to buy. Mary sitting in the front seat, had a glow about her as she talked about the house.

Willis Jr. and Monica were in the backseat of the car, and Mary turned and looked at them, asking if they liked the house. They both were smiling radiantly and almost laughing. They both said, "momma, I really like the house. Willis Jr. said, "The basement was large enough for him to roller-skate down there."

Monica told her mother, "I really liked my bedroom." Mary interrupted her, "Monica, I know just the furniture I am going to get for your bedroom. Baby, your bed will have "high bedposts with a fabric canopy over it, the same as a little princess would have. I'm going to get you a matching bedspread, and your dresser will have a mirror so you can see how pretty you look." Monica and Willis Jr. were excited about the house.

Even in jest, I made my standard comment to Mary. "Baby, there you go again, finding ways to spend money. The kids, Mary and I, laughed, and Willis Jr. and Monica cracked up. Monica said, "Daddy, Momma just wants to make the house look pretty, especially my room, " as she laughed louder."

I pulled up in front of my parents' house and parked the car. Willis Jr. and Monica ran to the front door, and I hollered, "don't knock on the door; I have a key to let us in." We went into the house, and my parents were in their favorite places, watching TV in the family room.

We said our hellos, and mother pampered and fussed over "Miss Renee," as she called Monica, who was sitting between her mother and grandmother on the couch. My dad was sitting in his recliner chair. I was sitting on the steps of the staircase, where I would always sit, and Willis Jr. was sitting by my side.

I was anxious to tell my parents about the first home that we were going to buy. I stood up, looked at my mom and dad, and said, "We just came from looking at the house we are going to buy. Mary, and the kids, really liked the house. It is in the price range that we can afford.

I believe this is the house we should buy and live in. Monica said, grandmamma, I like my bedroom. We all laughed. Mary said, "Mother Drake, it took a few trips to see the house again, and I really like the house."

I could see in my parent's faces that they were proud of Mary and me for being able to buy our first home. I was the youngest son, and I was 29 years old. I was their first child to buy a house among my seven siblings. At that moment, my entire family, Mary, and the kids were all beaming with joy.

Before I could say anymore, Mary excitedly started to describe the house. Mother said, "I have seen the house in a vision, and she described the house to the "T." In a declared fashion, she said, "Your family will not have any trouble living in that neighborhood when you move into your home."

Willis, before you move furniture or anything into your house. Take your Bible and form a circle holding hands with your wife and children. With the Bible in the center of the circle, you read the 23rd Psalm out loud to your family.

Mary and I had done our due diligence in consulting with our attorney to ensure that the house was sound construction-wise. Additionally, financially, Mary and I had sacrificed for over five years and saved our money wisely; to be in the best financial position to pay for our house outright. We knew we were truly blessed.

As was our normal routine, we prayed about buying the house that we felt was the house intended for us to own, and we decided to purchase the house. We were fortified in our decision with mother's words of encouragement and that she had seen us owning that house. We were confident this was the house for us to buy.

Mary and I met with our Easton and Taylor Trust Company Bank representative "Mr. Goodman," the bank's loan officer. With our personal savings account at the bank, we secured and guaranteed the mortgage loan. The financial arrangements with our Bank were swift and decisive. After finalizing the bank business, the purchase of our first home was imminent, and the transaction was completed.

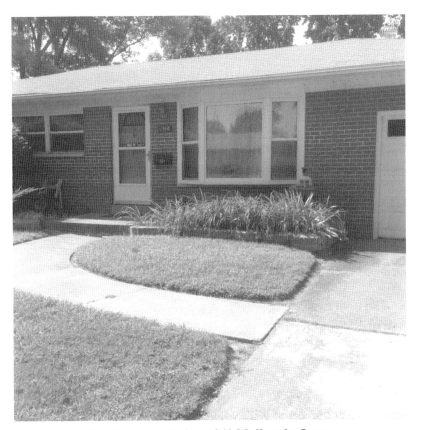

Our home located at:1340 Mullanphy Lane.

Naturally, as an African-American family, Mary and I had several concerns about potential problems our family might encounter moving into a primarily white environment. Most of all, we had concerns about how our two children, Willis Jr., and Monica (Kermit Matthew was not born yet), would be affected. Mary and I, as adults, could handle the overt and covert racism that we were sure we would encounter from some white people in our new community.

Growing up during the 1950s and 1960s in the St. Louis area, Mary and I experienced degrees of racism numerous times. Unfortunately, racism was ingrained among a considerable number of the white American population and perpetuated by them.

Our concern was for our young children and how they would cope with the "actual racist acts" they would likely encounter, at some level, living in this predominately white community. That was the issue Mary and I had to deal with. To this point in their lives, Mary and I had sheltered and protected our kids from direct hateful, and harmful racial experiences.

Living in Florissant potentially would be a totally new and possibly an unwelcomed harmful experience for both Willis Jr. at nine years old and Monica at seven years old regarding bigotry and hateful actions from racist individuals.

We had done the best job we knew how in raising and training our children to bring them up in the right way. Mary and I had instilled in our kids that they are capable of doing anything they put their minds to do.

Mary and I made the decision to purchase the house at 1340 Mullanphy Lane in Florissant, Missouri.

--- ◇ ---

CHAPTER 23

Memorial Day: Friday, May 30, 1969

--- ◇ ---

WITH THE HOUSE NOW PURCHASED, Mary was in very high spirits. Now the first thing she wanted to be done was to replace the carpets in the living room and dining room before we moved into the house.

My best friend Stan (Stanley McKissic) owned a floor-covering business. He had a business associate, Ronald (Ron), who owned a commercial and residential carpet business. Ironically, Ron lived in the 1300 block of Boulder Drive, exactly two blocks directly behind our house on Mullanphy Lane. He was a few years younger than Stan and me and a cool regular dude.

Mary selected a dark blue color carpet with an attractive embossed pattern design from Ron's carpet samples. The carpet was in stock, and Ron gave us a significant discount on the carpet price, re-arranged his work schedule, and installed the carpet in our house in two days.

Stan was the first person, friend, or family to see our new house. Stan and I were at the house while Ron and his worker installed the carpet. Meanwhile, day by day, in the evenings, Mary and I were packing up the apartment. Packing the boxes was more like fun than work. Willis

Jr. was helping me with the bulky items, and Monica was helping her mother with the small items to be packed.

Mary, the kids, and I moved most of our clothes and small household items during the week. Now we would move into our new house during the long three-day Memorial Day weekend, Friday, May 30, 1969. I only had to rent a U-Haul truck to move our furniture.

I picked up the U-Haul truck early Friday morning. I had help from family members and friends loading the furniture on the truck, and we were finished by noon. We would only need to make one trip to move our household belongings from the apartment to our new home.

Getting ready to leave the apartment, Willis Jr. said, "dad, I will miss going across the street to the park; that was always so much fun for me." With a genuine smile on my face, "I know, son, we were blessed living in this apartment." I closed and locked the door and got into the truck, and now we were heading to our new home in Florissant, Mo.

I drove cautiously as I entered interstate highway I-70 West. Mary was driving our car with the kids in the back seat. She was trailing behind the U-Haul truck going to the house.

We had been driving for 45 minutes when we came to Mullanphy Lane and headed to our new home, only five minutes away. Mary, the kids, and I got out of the vehicles, and I had our family bible in my hands. We followed my mother's spiritual guidance; we entered our house and formed a circle holding hands, and with our bible in the center, I read the 23rd Psalms aloud.

We started unloading the truck, and Mary had labels on each item indicating where it should go. We had purchased new furniture for the dining room, Monica's bedroom and a Chester-Drawer set for Willis Jr.'s bedroom that was being delivered by the furniture store later in the day.

Living at 1340 Mullanphy Lane, Florissant, MO

The U-Haul truck was now unloaded, and the furniture was in the place where Mary wanted it. I thanked everyone who helped us move and promised we would have a thank-you party soon for everyone who helped us move.

Mary and the kids followed me in our car to the U-Haul location, and I returned the truck and declared "mission accomplished." I was jubilant when I got in the car; Mary and the kids said, "it's time to get something to eat; we are hungry." Laughing, I said, "hey, I am hungry too.

We all had put in a full day's work getting us moved, and I know everybody was hungry." Mary said, "since you two worked so hard helping us move, you choose where we will go to eat."

Willis Jr. automatically shouted out let's go to McDonald's. Monica chimed in, agreeing wholeheartedly with her big brother, which was not often the case. Mary said, "okay, McDonald's it is," and we stopped at the McDonald's on Lindbergh that was close to our house. We were now ready to take our food and go back home to eat.

We pulled into our driveway within ten minutes of leaving McDonald's. Sitting in the car for a few seconds, I realized that the physical move was complete. Now there was an emotional sigh of relief, and we would spend the first night sleeping in our own house.

I opened the front door, and we went to the kitchen and put the food on the table. We washed up and sat at the kitchen table, and I blessed our food. We then ate our first meal, McDonald's hamburgers, French fries, and soda to drink in our new home together as a family.

When we were eating, Monica's effervescent laughter helped to ignite the lighthearted conversation we had at the dinner table. Mary and I heaped praise on Willis Jr. and Monica for being such a tremendous help getting us settled in our house. Now it was approaching the kid's bedtime, and our jovial conversation and McDonald's hamburgers had set the tone for the kids to have pleasant dreams sleeping the first night in our new home.

It was now close to 9:00 pm, and Willis Jr. and Monica were going to bed. Mary tiptoed barefoot across the living room to peep into the kids' rooms. Willis Jr.'s bedroom was directly across from our bedroom; Monica's bedroom was next to her brother's bedroom and slightly kitty-corner, across the hall from our bedroom.

Mary whispered and beckoned for me to come to the threshold of Monica's bedroom door as she was on her knees saying her prayers before getting in bed. We then observed Willis Jr. saying his prayers as he went to bed. We retreated to the living room, and we asked God to watch over our home and family in this new community.

For some reason, living in our new home felt unusual or just strange that first night. Maybe it was because we had lived seven years at 3715 Fair Avenue. Perhaps it was from my apprehension because we were an African-American family living in this predominantly white community.

What was vivid in my mind was that my Hi-Fi Stereo was unusually silent; I was stretched out on the couch, with my head on Mary's lap. I was relaxing and reflecting on our current life's journey. Looking up into Mary's eyes, "Baby, we stayed true to our plan, and we have been rewarded accordingly."

Now having enough money saved to pay for our house is a testament to God's blessings for us. Mary was smiling broadly, and she took my hand and led me from the couch as we retreated to the bedroom for the first night in our home. My thoughts were radiant as I acknowledged how truly blessed we were!

The Walk-Through With Mrs. Barnes

Mary and I had tidied up our old apartment, and on Saturday, the day after we had moved everything out of the apartment, we did a walk-thru with the owner, Mrs. Barnes. We returned her apartment keys to her and thanked her for trusting us, two young kids at that time, to take care of her property.

Mrs. Barnes expressed sadness in her voice, saying, "you young people were definitely the best tenants I have ever rented an apartment. Not once were you late in paying your rent. I am sorry to see us go, but buying your own home is tremendous progress for your young family."

She hugged Mary and me and wished us the best in our new home. As we were leaving the apartment, I reminded Mrs. Barnes what we promised her "If she rented us the apartment, we would take care of it and treat it as our home."

Mrs. Barnes smiling, said, "Yes, Mr. Drake, I remember well what you said, and you certainly did exactly that!" I said with pride to Mrs. Barnes, "My mother taught me that my word is my bond." Mary and I were determined to keep our "word" to you.

We had good friendly neighbors living at 3715 Fair Ave. The Wilson family lived in the apartment building next to the apartment building we lived in. The young boy was close to Willis Jr.'s age; his nickname was "Little Bit." I believe his name was Warren Wilson Jr., and he was two or three years older than Birdie.

Mary and I got along well with Little Bit's parents, and his older brother David was a really nice kid also. We never visited their apartment, and they didn't come into our apartment, but we were very good neighbors and socialized when we saw one another outside. No other children lived on the 3700 block of Fair Ave. at that time.

New Neighbors
We had lived in our home for a few days when our immediate neighbors, from next door and across the street, came to the house and introduced themselves to us. As Mary and I discussed the individual neighbors and their impromptu, or coordinated visit, it helped to allay the apprehension we assumed could happen to our family. Mary and I assessed that the neighbors' visits were a good-faith effort. Mary and I believe their

actions were intended as a "valid gesture" to our family, welcoming us to the neighborhood.

We appreciated the neighbor's friendliness in greeting our family to the community. It was significant because these neighbors were the parents of the kids (Schumacher and Hicks) that Willis Jr. and Monica were playing with in our backyard. It gave us confidence that our children were playing with kids from decent families.

Glenn Hicks's parents, Fred and Pauline Hicks were the first neighbors to come introduce themselves to Mary and me. They were an older couple in their early sixties. Mr. Hicks was a large man, about six feet tall and weighing over two hundred pounds. His wife Pauline was a woman of short stature, around five feet two inches tall, and weight-wise, she was on the chubby side.

They both worked for the Hazelwood School District; Mr. Hicks worked in the maintenance department, and Mrs. Hicks worked in the school's lunch (cafeteria) program department. Both Fred and Pauline Hicks were very friendly "Down-home" folks. Mary and I thought well of the Hicks, and they were good neighbors.

Mrs. Graham, a widow, and her seventeen years old son, Dale, a junior in high school, lived next door to the Hicks. Mr. Graham was deceased. He had retired as an officer in the United States Air Force. Mrs. Graham was a retired registered nurse in the United States Air Force.

That same week we moved into our house; Dale Graham, and a teenage friend of his, came to our house and introduced themselves. They wanted to know if we had teenage children their age, so they could meet them.

Each gesture of civility we received from our neighbors enhanced our belief that everything would be fine in our new home. Mrs. Graham was a petite, slightly built woman, weighing about 100 pounds and about five feet tall. She was a homemaker and apparently enjoyed baking desserts.

192

Gene and Anne Schumacher were Mary and Ronnie's parents, and they had seven children. Anne was a homemaker and Gene worked for the federal government at the Federal Aviation Administration (FAA) as a Supply Cataloger. They were good people, and they, too, welcomed our family to the neighborhood when we first moved into our house.

Our entire family, Mary, the kids, and I, had comfortably settled into our home that first weekend. Now it was June 2nd, and Willis Jr. and Monica would continue going to Eugene Field Elementary School for two weeks until their school year ended.

At our new house, our daily morning routine was for Mary to drop off Willis and Monica at mother's house so they could attend school. I also remember their last day of school and how emotional Willis Jr.'s teacher was that he was transferring to another school. She had raved about how smart he was and wanted to recommend him for special "exceptional accelerated school" for the coming school year.

Those two weeks in June passed quickly, and now we were comfortable in our new home. We were observing our immediate neighborhood to decide what our adult neighbors' attitudes and behavior would display. During the summer, a few months after we had moved into the neighborhood, a Chinese-American family, the Chins, moved next door to us.

Willis Jr. and Monica had made friends with the neighbor kids, the Schumacher's and Glenn Hicks, and now with the Chin family, they had an enjoyable, fun summer without any unpleasant incidents. As long as Willis Jr. and Monica had friends to play with on an equal and acceptable basis, that was what mattered to Mary and me.

However, neither Mary nor I reached out to our adult neighbors sociably, as we had our own social life established within our circle of friends, family, and culture. However, we were cordial and responsive to our neighbors reaching out to us.

Often Mrs. Graham would bring Mary cookies and pastries she had just baked. From their first meeting, with Mary also being a nurse, she and

Mrs. Graham appeared to have connected well with one another. Periodically they had pleasant conversations as Mrs. Graham would come to the house and talk to Mary.

Mrs. Graham also was the person that knew just about everything happening in the immediate neighborhood. She would ring the doorbell, and with the plate of goodies in hand, Mary would invite her into the house. Mary knew the desserts were Mrs. Graham's cover, so she could share the current neighborhood news with Mary.

Mary considered Mrs. Graham visiting the house a social visit. The common thread that they had was the nursing profession. They enjoyed one another's company, laughing and absorbing the tidbits of information shared, and Mary enjoyed the visits from Mrs. Graham tremendously.

At night before we went to sleep, Mary's eyes would light up, and she enjoyed regurgitating the conversations she and Mrs. Graham had earlier in the day. That social exchange between Mrs. Graham and Mary constituted a level of comfort and, sort of, a welcome to the neighborhood. In just a brief time, only weeks, our family was feeling overall more at ease about our new neighborhood.

Thankfully, none of the horrendous racist situations reported in other surrounding St. Louis communities didn't occur in our immediate neighborhood. However, school would be starting in a month, and Willis Jr. and Monica would be exposed to a broader population of kids in the overall community.

CHAPTER 24

Children—McCurdy Elementary School

I T APPEARED ALMOST MYTHICAL THAT September was right around the corner. Willis Jr. and Monica had enjoyed a fun summer in our new home. Mary and I were extremely encouraged by our family's reception from our neighbors during the summer months.

Now Labor Day, September 7, 1969, was approaching, and the kids would be attending McCurdy Elementary School in the Hazelwood School District. Their school was located at 975 Lindsay Lane, Florissant, MO 63031, only four short blocks from our house.

Despite the short distance of four blocks to walk to school, we still felt the "dry run" was necessary, regardless of the distance to school. To get ready for school, in mid-August, Mary and I walked with eight years old Willis Jr. and six years old Monica along the neighborhood streets, showing them the route to take in walking to and from school.

We were methodical in our instructions and directions for them to walk to school. We started from our house on Mullanphy Lane. They walked one-third of a block (two houses) to Loveland Lane, and they would turn left. The first street they would cross was Aspen Drive. They would turn right on the next street, Boulder Drive. They would turn right on the next street, Manor Drive. They would cross the next street, Estes Drive. They would continue walking for one block to get to Lindsay Lane, and they would turn left, and McCurdy Elementary school was located at 975 Lindsay Lane.

Over the summer, our family had assimilated into the neighborhood comfortably. Willis Jr. and Monica had made friends with the immediate neighbors' kids. Those friendships were effectively in a bubble, encapsulating a few families living next-door and across the street from our house.

The days were fast approaching, which caused Mary and I to scrutinize the broader community when school would start. Our concern was if that "comfortable bubble" would literally burst. Willis Jr. was a third-grader, and Monica was in the first grade. Mary and I were concerned about how we could protect our kids "from verbal hostility" when exposed to a broader population of kids in the school community.

We emphasized to our kids not to deviate from this route walking to and from school. We didn't want to put fear in their minds from just walking to school. However, we wanted a pattern they would follow in case we needed to retrace the route they walked, going to and from school. As African-American parents in this community, we were not certain what racial attitudes our children would face at school in general. Therefore we felt precautions are better than the "I wish I could've, would've, or should've" Syndrome.

The McCurdy Elementary School principal was apparently guided by some "force or motivation" to meet our family before school started.

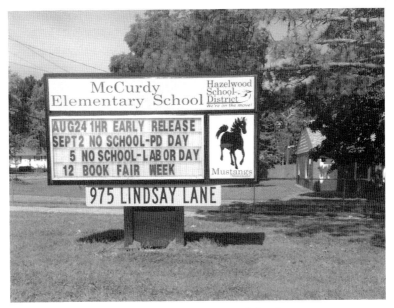

McCurdy Elementary School

Mr. Gerald Gilmer, the principal at McCurdy Elementary School, had stopped at our neighbor, Mr. Hicks' house, on a few occasions during the summer. I was cutting my front lawn in early August when Fred Hicks and Mr. Gilmer walked across the front lawn to our house.

Mr. Hicks was an affable person; as usual, he always smiled when we talked. He wore his bibbed overalls with a T-shirt underneath. The man with him wore a casual short sleeve sports shirt and slacks.

Hello, Mr. Drake, "I want to introduce you to Mr. Gerald Gilmer. He is the principal at McCurdy Elementary School, where Willis and Monica will be attending. Your family being new to the school, Mr. Gilmer wanted to meet you before school starts.

Quickly I observed that Mr. Gilmer was about five feet, seven or eight inches tall; average weight for his height; he wore eyeglasses and had mingled gray hair, and he had a personable smile. He said, "Hello, Mr. Drake," as he extended his right hand. We shook hands, and I returned his greeting.

We exchanged a few pleasantries, and he "saw that your children will be attending McCurdy Elementary School." Therefore, he asked Fred to introduce us. He appeared to be a very pleasant man, stating, "He hope our family was adjusting to the neighborhood well."

I confirmed, "Yes, our family had adjusted well to the community, thankfully because of our neighbors like Mr. Hicks' family. It did not escape me that there was a real concern in the school's principal mind that my children might encounter some unpleasant situations when they started school. Otherwise, I don't think Mr. Gilmer would want to meet me prior to school starting. He apparently recognized that potential problems could exist, the same as I had.

We talked for fifteen minutes, and as he was leaving, Mr. Gilmer said, "Mr. Drake let me know if you or your children have any problems at the school. That initial introduction was the first of many future conversations that Gerald Gilmer, Mary, and I would have over the next several years. Mr. Gilmer proved to be a very fair-minded man and an advocate of progressive change.

As it turned out, Mr. Gilmer coming to my home to introduce himself was significant, in the broadest sense, to aid our family in adjusting to the overall McCurdy Elementary School environment.

African-American Families Living in the Community
When we moved into the neighborhood, two African-American families lived in the community; only one family had children attending McCurdy Elementary School. The one family lived on Mullanphy Lane, two blocks north of our house. Their son Jay was a few years older than Willis Jr., and he would visit his dad during the summer, but he lived with his mother in California, where he attended school.

The other African-American family in the community lived three blocks from our house on one of the side streets off Mullanphy Lane. When school started and as time passed, Mary would talk with the mother frequently (Cookie is the only name I recall she used). I tried ad nauseam to establish a relationship with the father but to no avail. Based on

Mary's conversations with Cookie, she believes they were foster care parents. They had three Elementary school-age children living in the house with them.

Their family had lived in the neighborhood, and their kids had attended McCurdy Elementary School for the full school year. In talking with Mary, Cookie sometimes would describe the attitudes of the "white parents" at McCurdy School, in general, as not friendly. Periodically Willis Jr. and Monica would visit Cookie's children at their home after school.

When African-Americans moved into a predominantly white neighborhood, it was not unusual, albeit biased or prejudicial. Those African-American families were heavily scrutinized by their white neighbors. As a rule, the white residents living in the neighborhood often prejudge African American families. Regardless if they had met the family or not, and certainly they did not know these African-American families from a single or a few encounters.

It was routine that white residents would examine actions taken by African-American families living in the community from afar. Some white families would criticize directly or indirectly these African-American families as being strange, unusual, or improperly behaving. Perhaps it was based on if these actions or habits were not consistent with their white "cultural" experience. I believe that our family's every move initially underwent that same scrutiny from our neighbors.

However, I know our family just lived the way that was "who we were." We did not try to impress our neighbors. We were just reflecting on who we were and our true character as decent human beings. Our actions reflected the beliefs and teachings (the culture) with which we were raised.

As congenial and friendly as the kids living next door and across the street from us were. Conversely, there were two older white boys that also went to McCurdy Elementary School that tried to physically bully my kids. Going to and coming from school, they called them the racial slur "N" word.

I had told Willis Jr. and Monica to ignore anyone that called them names and to come home and let me know what happened. However, don't you just let anyone "mess over you, okay? You protect yourself and fight back if you must!"

Mr. Gilmer, McCurdy Elementary School Principal
Following that first name-calling incident, Mary and I went to school the next day, met with Mr. Gilmer, and discussed the issue. He was apologetic and assured us that if Willis Jr. and Monica had any more problems during the school day, have them report it to their teacher or him immediately.

He stressed that Mr. and Mrs. Drake, "I don't condone that name-calling, and be assured that I will definitely address this situation. Fortunately, as Willis and Monica got established in McCurdy Elementary School, those situations did not continue.

Moreover, unfortunately, some McCurdy Elementary School staff teachers were polluted with their own biases and prejudices. As parents, Mary and I were still assessing how Willis Jr. and Monica were adjusting to the McCurdy School. However, we would soon realize that the adjustment needed should be directed more so to some of the McCurdy Elementary School teachers themselves.

Monica's teacher also had a daughter (Cindy) in Willis's third-grade class. As usual, every evening at the dinner table, Mary and I would encourage Willis Jr. and Monica to tell us how their day was at school. We would discreetly ask questions to get as much information as we could from them.

In late September, during our dinner discussion, Monica was excited as she told us, "Her school class picture day will be in two weeks. Momma, my teacher said we should wear something "nice" for picture day." With her bright smile and animated gestures, Monica said, "We will have our class picture, but I will also have an individual picture by myself."

Mary smiled and said, "Monica, I will make you a special pretty dress for your picture day, okay." Looking at Mary, I thought she was a chip off the old block. Mary's mother was a terrific seamstress, and she would make Mary special outfits when she was in elementary school.

Through her innate ability, or genuine interest, and what her mother had taught her, Mary had learned how to lay out sewing patterns and to sew practically any clothing design. Now, as an adult, with a professional career, Mary only sewed occasionally. She had a modern upscale sewing machine and enjoyed sewing when she had the time.

In the following days, Mary and Monica looked at pictures in children's magazines of dresses for little girls. With meticulous creativity, Mary had transformed that bright yellow fabric she had bought into this beautiful dress for Monica to wear for her school photo day.

On the morning of Monica's school picture day, Mary dressed her in the beautiful yellow dress with brown trimmings she had made. Before I left for work, I marveled over how pretty Monica looked in her dress. I told her she looked beautiful, just like a "Little Princess."

That evening at the dinner table, Monica was speaking in a monotone voice. She said, "momma, during "show-and-tell," I told my classmates that you made my dress, and "my dad said," I look like a beautiful Little Princess."

Monica said, "After I did my show and tell, my teacher had me stand in front of the classroom and said, "Class do you think Monica looks like a princess?" She didn't do that with the other (white) students. Momma, I felt awkward standing in front of the class like that."

I could see the veins in Mary's neck protruding, and she said, "okay, baby, you should not feel uncomfortable in your classroom for any reason. I will go to the school to talk with your teacher.

Hearing what Monica's teacher had done, Mary and I both were ticked-off, but we quenched our anger in front of the kids. I reaffirmed to Monica that she truly looked like a beautiful little princess in her beautiful dress this morning. Looking at Mary, I could tell that she was seething and wanted to get that teacher straightened out quickly.

As we finished eating dinner, Mary hugged Monica, and they started cleaning up the dinner dishes.

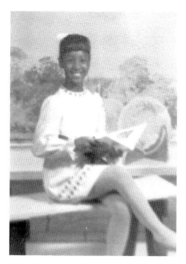

Monica on school picture day

That night Mary and I seriously discussed how we would handle the situation with Monica's teacher. The teacher obviously had a propensity for displaying racist behavior, and she evidently wanted to make a spectacle of Monica, the only African-American child in her classroom. In the teacher's racist mind, she could not envision how Monica could look like a beautiful princess.

I could imagine the thoughts running through that teacher's mind. She had to be thinking "The audacity of Monica's father, telling his daughter that she was beautiful and looked like a princess. The nerve of that man telling his daughter she is beautiful."

Before we could confront Monica's teacher regarding the photo incident, a second situation happened within days of the first incident. Monica told us "that her teacher had passed out candy treats to the class, and she only gave her licorice (black) jellybeans. She told Monica, "I know you like these jellybeans, " implying that because Monica was African-American, she liked the licorice jellybeans.

I had not ever seen Mary that angry before, never! Later that evening, she said, "Willis, I am going to the school tomorrow to see Monica's teacher. I thought the first picture day incident was an aberration, but now, the teacher has shown her true racism as clearly as she can."

I asked Mary if she wanted me to go to the school with her. "No, no, baby, I will take care of this alone, she responded. The proclivity of Monica's teacher's spiteful covert racial behavior prompted Mary to go to school the next day and have a very convincing "heart-to-heart" woman-to-woman conversation with the teacher.

In their meeting, Mary asked the teacher directly if she had a problem because Monica is African American. She vehemently denied being biased toward Monica. Mary described her conversation with the teacher as forceful in her tone and words. "Willis, I made it clear that she was not to single out Monica in front of the classroom again for any reason."

After Mary had her conversation with Monica's teacher, that teacher's improper behavior ceased; at least she didn't single out Monica again. Mary let it be known that if any incident occurred again, her next step would be to formally address the issue with the school's administration. Mary and I followed up her meeting with the teacher with a meeting with Mr. Gilmer to address this situation.

Periodically, Mary and I would have a casual conversation with Mr. Gilmer, the principal. At every opportunity, he would recommend that we become active with the Parents' Teachers Association (PTA) and other auxiliary parents groups. We joined the PTA, and Mary was active with the organization, as most of the members were the students' mothers.

The president of the PTA was a young, intelligent, fair-minded mother of two students at the school, and her son was in Willis' class. She seemly influenced or at least guided the members of the PTA to her thought processes. Mary brought a sense of independence to the group.

The president of the PTA and Mary connected with an appreciable level of continuity in their opinions.

As the school year positively progressed, Mr. Gilmer was discretely keeping an eye on Willis Jr. and Monica. With Mary and me reflecting on our authentic natural character, it apparently made a favorable impression on Mr. Gilmer. Unpretentiously, our family provided an image that reflected the reality that our kids were normal, intelligent, and well-capable as any other student in their class.

As Willis Jr. and Monica's parents, we were involved in school activities that required our normal participation. We were involved at the same level of participation that the other student's parents were in the school's activities. We supported our children's educational goals and school activities, as well as any other parents in the school.

Mr. Gilmer, Mary, and I had several meaningful conversations throughout the school year. We talked about specific attitudes that were germane to the McCurdy School. Without a doubt, from our perspective, Mary and I felt there were several teachers at the school that displayed subtle racial bias tendencies.

It was interesting that Mr. Gilmer shared with us his plans for the next school semester at McCurdy Elementary. It was pleasantly surprising when he stated, "for a few years now, I have wanted to hire an African-American teacher at McCurdy School."

However, in some form, his staff had expressed opposition when he indicated he was considering hiring an African-American teacher. There always was a negative pushback from a small segment of the teachers. Mr. Gilmer was basically isolated with the idea of hiring an African-American teacher.

Seeing the emotion on his face, it was obvious to me that this was something he was committed to doing. He said, "Mr. and Mrs. Drake, your family has given me the example that I can now point to if I get any negative comments or pushback from my teachers and staff.

"I will hire an African-American teacher at McCurdy Elementary School starting the next school year in September."

I am unsure if Mr. Gilmer had any expectations of our family or if he had anticipated how we would be involved in the McCurdy Elementary School. I knew that Willis Jr. and Monica were intelligent, they knew they could accomplish anything they put their mind to doing, and they were raised with proper upbringing and the right values. They would not be outliers in the school.

Mary and I knew that our children would measure up equally to their classmates in every regard. Personality-wise, they were very likable kids, especially Willis Jr., with his outgoing personality; his classmates were attracted to him like a magnet to metal.

Personally, I had a slight advantage compared to some families that had children attending McCurdy School. My former coworkers at the Mart Building and my current coworkers at the Mobility Equipment Command, that lived in Florissant, had children attending McCurdy Elementary School and other schools in the Hazelwood school district.

Therefore, I could look the parents of my children's classmates in their eyes; because I was cognizant of their behavior on the job at work. I knew who their friends were or who they fraternized with.

Also, they knew that their wives or husbands were not any more educated, technically trained, or professionally astute than Mary and I were. Their children generally were not anymore intelligent or gifted as our children were.

So, it was quite easy to understand that I was not in awe of my neighbors in my new Florissant community. I knew that my wife, children, and I belonged in this community and any community where we could afford to live.

Mr. Gilmer, true to his word, over the summer hired Mrs. Dorothy Payne, and she was one of the first African-American teachers in the Hazelwood school system. Interestingly enough, she was my daughter Monica's second-grade teacher. Following Monica's negative experience with her first-grade teacher's subtle racist attitude, Mrs. Payne was an inspiration and role model that Monica could look up to.

Because Mrs. Payne was Monica's teacher, Mary and I had several conversations with her as parents during the students' conferences. As well as African-Americans in the same generation reflected common experiences that were very revealing. Mrs. Payne told us of the negative reactions she initially received from the McCurdy Elementary School's teaching staff when she was hired. That some of the teachers, passing her in the hallway, would turn their heads so they would not have to speak to her.

Mrs. Payne also commented on the tremendous support she received from McCurdy Elementary School principal, Mr. Gilmer. She said that he was a terrific principal and a friend also, and she witnessed, due to Mr. Gilmer's leadership, the change in the attitudes of the overall teaching staff at McCurdy School over the years.

Mrs. Payne's comments about Monica's first-grade teacher confirmed further what Mary and I had already discerned about that teacher. She was racist to the extent that she would not afford Mrs. Payne the human decency, or the professional courtesy, as a coworker and fellow teacher to speak to her as an equal when passing her in the McCurdy Elementary School's hallways.

Years later, I contacted Mrs. Payne, and she revealed further about her experiences when she first started teaching at McCurdy School. Also, we were laughing when she said that "The teacher (Monica's first-grade teacher) that would not say hello to her initially walking in the hallways at school, had sent her a "Friend me invitation on Facebook" after she retired and moved to Florida. Mrs. Payne said I didn't respond. We both just had a hearty laugh.

As "humans," sometimes we must understand and accept that there is a "Power greater than we are" that intercedes and guides us to make the right decisions. Some people may call it intuition, a gut feeling, but I recognized it as the Holy Spirit. I know the house at 1340 Mullanphy Lane we purchased was intended for us. As a result, we as a family would be fine living in our house. Moreover, our children, Willis Jr. and Monica, would overcome any adverse racist attitudes they encountered at school as well.

CHAPTER 25

---◇---

Willis Jr. Music Ability

---◇---

Entering the fourth grade, students could join the McCurdy Elementary School band. Starting his second year at McCurdy School, Willis Jr. was nine years old, going into the fourth grade.

Still, today, I remember vividly that evening as if it was yesterday. For some reason, which was unusual, Mary had arrived home before me. When I got home from work, Mary was in the kitchen preparing dinner. Willis Jr. met me at the front door and gave me a man hug.

I had not seen him this animated in quite some time, although he could be overly dramatic at times. He smiled and said, " Dad, can I join the school band? I want to play the trumpet like Louis Armstrong."

I had to maneuver my way in the front door to get pass Willis Jr. I was now smiling, hearing my son say he wanted to play the trumpet like Louis Armstrong, or maybe because my workday was over and I was glad to be home. It was great that he had an African-American musician trumpet player, Louis Armstrong, to inspire him.

However, my favorite trumpet player was Miles Davis, and I had record albums of Miles and Satchmo that I played in our home often. However,

I did not realize Willis Jr. was listening or paying attention to Louis Armstrong's music.

Laughing as I was now inside the house, "Son, slow down. Anyway, what do you know about "Satchmo." We both laughed, and he said, "dad, I hear his record albums that you play on your Hi-Fi, and I've seen Satchmo on TV. I know about him! Can I join the school band and play the trumpet?"

I had a reflective moment thinking that continuing to expose our kids to their cultural background, overall was registering with them. In their current environment, it was especially important for them to be in touch with their African-American history. Living in a predominately white community and school system, African-American history was not emphasized, if taught at all.

Walking towards the kitchen, Willis was beside me, hanging onto my arm. "Did you ask your mother if you could join the band?" He quickly said yes, and mom told me to ask you. I was now in the kitchen, and I kissed Mary. I asked her what do you think, babe. She looked at Willis Jr. "Birdie, as long as you can keep up your grades in your regular schoolwork, I think it will be okay to join the school band."

I said, "Okay Willis, you know my rule. "If you start anything, particularly playing the trumpet, you will have to stick with it. That means you will practice every day, regardless if you want to go outside and play with Glen and Ronnie. You will have to practice your trumpet, and you heard what your mother said about your school grades."

Half laughing, Birdie said okay, dad, it is a deal; let's shake on it. That was how my son and I sealed our "word to one another."

I signed the authorization agreement so Birdie could participate in the McCurdy School band. We had the option to lease or purchase the trumpet, and we chose to purchase it for him. That commitment made it clear that he would stick with learning to play the trumpet.

His gift of music was instantaneous. Within two or three weeks, Willis Jr. was playing simple songs on his trumpet, such as "The Three Blind Mice, Twinkle Twinkle Little Star, and Mary Had A Little Lamb." By the second month, Willis Jr.'s progress allowed him to play songs from sheet music the band instructor had given him to practice. He also would practice for one full hour each day during the week. His weekend practices were voluntary, but he sometimes practiced on weekends.

The song "Born Free" was still popular during that year. Willis would turn ten years old in November 1970. He had only been playing the trumpet for a few months. He had always been a big "Ham," and it did not take much encouragement for him to be on center stage.

The McCurdy school's band instructor had requested permission from the school's principal, Mr. Gilmer, to have the students come outside on the grounds to hear Willis Jr. play the song Born Free. Being the natural "Ham," he played the song flawlessly.

After he had played his trumpet solo for the McCurdy School, he was the talk of the school and the broader neighborhood community. At the time, we attended a local church, Florissant Presbyterian Church, in the Florissant area. The church pastor, Rev. Stewart, had initially come by our house with his wife and welcomed us to the community.

Subsequently, he had heard from members of the church's congregation how Willis played the trumpet, and Rev. Stewart asked me if Willis Jr. could play his trumpet during a church service, which he did. When we visited our parents, he would naturally play his trumpet for his grandparents.

During the McCurdy Elementary School Parents Teacher's Conference, the band instructor asked Mary and me if we could "get Willis private music lessons as soon as possible. He stated that "Willis has a musical gift that he had not seen at such a young age, and it should be cultivated."

I asked the band instructor, "If he knows where I could get private trumpet lessons for Willis?" He referred us to a local music store in the area, where college students majoring in music were the music instructors. They came highly recommended by the colleges and were very good musicians.

I contacted the music store owner and scheduled an appointment with the trumpet instructor for private trumpet lessons for Willis Jr. The trumpet lessons were confirmed at the music store, one day a week, and the music session would last an hour.

Willis Jr. and I arrived at the music store Tuesday at 5:30 pm. The man behind the display counter asked if he could help us. I told him, "My son had an appointment for his first trumpet lesson with a music instructor."

He introduced himself as the owner of the music store, and he paged the music instructor on the PA system. In minutes, the trumpet instructor was at the front counter, and he introduced himself to me and Willis Jr. He was about twenty-one years old, a college student in his junior year, and majoring in music. He also played the trumpet as his primary musical instrument.

I stayed at the music store while Willis Jr. was having his music lesson. Only a half-hour had passed, and I saw Willis Jr. and the young trumpet instructor walking up the aisle toward the front of the store. They were talking and sort of laughing as they reached me. I was surprised to see them return that soon. Willis' music lesson was scheduled for an hour.

The young music teacher said, "Mr. Drake, your son Willis, has tremendous musical ability, and I am sorry; there is nothing I can teach him. You will need to get a music teacher that's much better than I am to give him trumpet lessons." The music instructor put his hand on Willis' shoulder and said, "Man, I know you are going to be awesome, and I hope you get a teacher that can help you advance musically in playing the trumpet."

When we got home, I told Mary what the young trumpet teacher had said. She was as surprised as I was regarding Willis' music potential. We both knew Willis played the trumpet well from listening to him practice.

Mary and I agreed we would find a qualified music teacher to give Birdie trumpet lessons.

I talked with Willis' band director for other recommendations for getting Willis Jr. trumpet lessons. Unfortunately, he did not know anyone in the immediate Florissant County area to recommend. I used the local telephone directory and contacted a music teacher in Dellwood, a city in north St. Louis County. It was a considerable distance, about 45 minutes from our home.

During our initial telephone conversation, the music teacher said he did not give lessons to children as young as Willis Jr. He suggested I find a music teacher that gave trumpet lessons to elementary school-age children my son's age. I amplified the best I could "that I had exhausted all means to find a teacher in my area to give my son trumpet lessons. You are the only music instructor I found near where we live."

The music teacher said, "Children had to be more musically advanced than a ten-year-old would be for him to give music lessons. That his music training was designed to teach classical music theory, reading, and playing from sheet music." He emphasized, "If a musician could learn to play classical music, then a classical musician can play all other types of music."

The instructor (I do not recall his name) said, "I will give your son one music lesson to see if I can recommend someone to give him trumpet lessons."

He informed me that the cost was twenty dollars for him to listen and evaluate where my son was musically. That was the same cost he charged for a one-hour music lesson. In effect, it was an audition to see if Willis Jr. could get a music instructor to give him trumpet lessons.

The following Tuesday, Willis Jr. and I were in the car driving to the music studio; consequentially, I cautioned him not to be disappointed if the music teacher could not give him trumpet lessons. However, he might be able to recommend a particularly good music teacher for him.

We had been driving for half an hour, and I was not familiar with the area. I think it was on West Florissant Road. The studio was located in a "Strip Mall," and only eight or ten businesses were located there. I pulled into the mall area and parked in front of this two-story building. The music studio was upstairs on the second floor.

When we got to the small lobby area (waiting room), the music teacher came to meet us. He only had a few words to say to me as he formally introduced himself, and we shook hands. Then he asked Willis Jr. to come with him so he could hear him play his trumpet.

I remained in the waiting room, and an hour later, they returned, and the music instructor said, "Mr. Drake, your son, Willis, shows an enormous amount of musical ability, and potential, for only having played the trumpet for a few months. He is more advanced than some of the students I have been giving trumpet lessons to for several years.

I am excited to have Willis as a student, and his trumpet lessons will be Tuesdays at 6:00 o'clock every week." Willis' musical ability was being transformed exponentially as he received trumpet lessons from his music instructor. Willis received music lessons from his trumpet instructor for the next four years until we moved from Florissant to Battle Creek, Michigan, in 1974.

Willis' music teacher expressed regretful disappointment to see Willis Jr. move from the area. Because he was now seeing the benefits from the past four years that he has been teaching Willis Jr. to play the trumpet more expertly like a classical trumpet player. The music instructor said he was sorry that he would not be able to continue to work with him.

The music instructor said, "The music talent that Willis has displayed only comes along every now and then. Mr. Drake, be sure to get Willis a music instructor that will motivate and keep pushing him forward.

As I reflect and analyze our move to Battle Creek, I also must recognize what may have been restrictions or a negative impact on the development of Willis Jr.'s' music advancement. There was no music instructor in the Battle Creek area to help advance Willis' musical ability.

Willis' Springfield Junior High and Senior High School band teacher, Mr. Strickland, was a strong supporter of Willis. He registered him in various high school music competitions at the district and state levels. Willis Jr. excelled in individual music competitions and was highly recognized for his achievements in playing the trumpet.

Willis as a Springfield high school band member, was selected to participate in the at large combined Michigan Lions Club (MLC) high school band. As a member of this band he traveled to Tokyo, Japan, one year and the next year he traveled to Canada, performing with the MLC band.

From the very first time Willis Jr. picked up the trumpet as a fourth-grader at McCurdy Elementary school, it was as if he was born to play that musical instrument. He had an extraordinary musical propensity and God-given talent to play the trumpet naturally.

CHAPTER 26

$\diamondsuit$

Mary Wants Another Baby

$\diamondsuit$

MARY AND I HAD BEEN married for nine years when we bought our first house. We had an eight-year-old son and a six-year-old daughter. Everything had fallen in place in accordance with our (my) plan, which would allow us to pay off our twenty-year house mortgage in three years, and we would be debt free.

We had initiated and executed our plan for the future extraordinarily well. We would own our house outright, and we had established the kid's college fund quite sufficiently. My long-term strategy was being executed as I had planned. I saw our opportunity to secure financial security for our family as ideal.

However, Mary had her desires, and she wanted to have another baby, a girl, or a boy; it didn't matter. We discussed the pros and cons of expanding our family. I reminded her that Willis Jr. and Monica were approaching the age where they could do so much for themselves now and that being a parent would be much easier.

With that pretty smile and sensual look on her face, Mary beckoned for me to come closer. She embraced me and whispered, "Willis, it will be so nice to have another baby." Mary was influencing my mindset to have another baby. When Willis Jr. was born, we were young kids, Mary was nineteen, and I was twenty. Two years later, Monica was born, and neither of their births was "planned."

Mary and I decided we would have another baby in 1970. At age twenty-nine, she would enjoy the experience of motherhood from a different perspective. When Mary confirmed that she was pregnant, we both were extremely happy. As her pregnancy advanced, it was exciting when I would rub her stomach and feel the baby's heartbeat. That made me act like a new nervous, expecting dad all over again.

Looking at Mary, it was difficult to tell that she was four months pregnant. She planned a social gathering at our home on Saturday evening to announce we were expecting a baby later this year. We invited family members and our closest friends to our house party. Willis Jr. and Monica spent that weekend at their grandmother Ruby's house in East St. Louis.

The guests started arriving at 8:00 pm, and Mary was putting her final touches on the food and refreshments she was preparing. I was circulating between upstairs, answering the door, and in the basement, ensuring our guests were comfortable.

When the last guests arrived, and everybody was in the rathskeller, Mary descended the steps to the basement rathskeller with a tray of Hors-d'oeuvres in her hands.

She was wearing a black and white checkered maternity top and black pants. Her face was radiant and it seemed to illuminate the basement. Mary's closest friend Vickie (Virginia Vaughn) was surprised to see Mary in a maternity outfit. She quickly took the tray of hors d'oeuvres from Mary's hands and hugged her.

Vickie was animated, exclaiming, "Mary, girl, why didn't you tell me you are expecting?" Then the other ladies and everybody hugged and congratulated Mary and me. The traditional question of when is the baby due was echoed repeatedly by the ladies with excitement.

The gaiety continued, and in the midst of all of the joy and congratulations, I had my arms around Mary's waist, and we thanked our family and friends for sharing in our blessed announcement that our baby would be due in November this year (1970).

The night ended with Mary and me straightening up the basement, putting away leftover food, and loading the dishes in the dishwasher. As we were getting ready for bed, Mary was still excited about the announcement to our friends that we were having a baby in six months.

Sunday morning, when we woke up, we went to get the kids. Mary was still beaming as she described to her mother how our friends reacted to the news that she is expecting a baby in November.

Mrs. Byas, with her sense of humor was laughing and said, "Pookie, it had been eight years since you had a baby in the house. So get ready for the midnight feeding and everything with a new baby.

Monica was bubbling over and said, "Grandmamma Ruby, I will help momma take care of the baby." Laughing, she hugged her granddaughter, saying, "Monica, I know you will be a big help to your mother, just like you are when you are here with me." We got ready to leave, and we said our goodbyes.

Driving home, Willis Jr. and Monica debated if their mother was going to have a girl or a boy. Each of them rationalized why they wanted a baby sister or baby brother. Mary chimed in, saying we will have to wait and see if it will be a boy or girl, but we just want a healthy baby, okay? We arrived home, and our routine was normal.

As time passed, the weeks led into months, and Mary was having a normal pregnancy, and there were no issues health-wise. We had all the necessary scenarios in place for when the baby was born. We decided if the baby was a girl, we would name her Ruby Dean Drake, after Mary's mother's first name and my mother's middle name. If the baby was a boy, we would name him Kermit Matthew Drake, after my father's first name and Mary's father's first name, as the baby's middle name.

The final result was manifested 19 months after we had moved into the first home we had bought. Our son Kermit Matthew Drake was born at St. Luke's Hospital, in St. Louis, Mo., at 5:00 pm, on Thursday, November 19, 1970. Kermit's birth was truly a blessing to Mary and me, just the same as Willis Jr. and Monica were.

When I brought Mary and Kermit Matthew home, it was gratifying to see the reception from our neighbors. They brought gifts for the baby and welcomed Mary and Kermit Matthew home. With the reaction to our family, I recognized that we really had good neighbors.

It didn't take Mary any time to glide into being the mother of an infant baby again. The early morning or late-night feedings and diaper changes were routine. I did my share of changing diapers and early morning feedings too.

Growing up, Mary never learned to swim. I learned to swim when I was 12 years old at Tandy Center after my friends threw me in the shadow water of the (indoor) swimming pool. I did not have a swimming instructor; my lesson was "sink or swim." Swimming customary is not commonly part of the African-American cultural experiences. When Kermit was six or seven months old, Mary enrolled him in a "water baby swimming class" so he could learn to swim as a baby.

Mary would take Kermit to his swimming classes twice a week, and a parent had to be in the swimming pool with their child. Mary was a willing participant in the shadow end of the swimming pool, where the water was three feet deep.

After his swim lesson, Mary was so excited describing how Kermit had swum. Mary's face would light up, and I would humor her, saying, "baby, I know Kermit can't swim at nine months old. She was adamant as she proclaimed, Willis, you will have to come see him. He swims like a little fish."

I went to Kermit's swimming classes, and sure enough, he could swim at the age of 9 months. Ironically, Willis Jr. and Monica learned to swim during summer camp when they were six or seven years old.

Mary did not work when Kermit was a baby; she was a full-time stay-at-home mom. This was totally different from when Willis Jr. and Monica were babies; Mary was attending nursing school. Notwithstanding being a full-time nursing student, Mary was a terrific mother to Willis Jr. and Monica. Our kids, Willis Jr., Monica, and Kermit Matthew, were truly blessed and fortunate to have Mary as their mother.

When Kermit turned two years old, Mary decided she wanted to work part-time on weekends. She got a job immediately at the St. Louis Jewish Hospital, working in the psychiatric department. Working weekends was sufficient to reinvigorate her professional urge for being a nurse again, and she was able to hone her nursing skills with current nursing information and practices.

Moreover, Mary enjoyed getting outside the house and engaging her nursing colleagues at work. Working the weekends also allowed her to interact with adult nursing professionals, which was mentally and intellectually stimulating for her. However, she remained exuberant in taking care of her baby, Kermit.

Kermit was the Kingpin in the household, particularly on the weekends. His big sister Monica would coddle his every need and reaction. At eight years old, she was his surrogate mother, babying him on all occasions. Between Monica and next-door neighbor Patty Chin, Kermit ruled our backyard as the youngest baby in the circle of the neighboring family friends.

Then occasionally, our neighbor across the street, Monica Schumacher, who was five or six years old, would join in favoring Kermit while playing in our backyard. On the other hand, at 12 years old, Willis Jr. played the rough big brother role with Kermit to make him tougher than a two-year-older should be.

On the weekends, when Willis Jr. and Monica had their weekend sports activities, Kermit was always with me at their practices and ball games. The mothers of their teammates would also offer to hold Kermit and look after him at the ball field so I could get involved in the games like the other dads.

I was able to hold down the "home front" on the weekends very well. I cared for the kids; however, Willis Jr. and Monica were responsible kids and did not require much attention. I took care of Kermit, and Monica was an immense help to me in caring for him.

Working the weekends gave Mary a break from her daily household responsibilities of caring for the kids for a brief time. She also could engage in learning the new and updated nursing practices being used in a progressive St. Louis Jewish Hospital institution.

Mary arrived home one night, and she was in a talking mood. She said, "Willis, I have come through; rather, we have come through challenges that many young people our age never survive. I know we are blessed. I am able to be home during the week with our children, and on the week-ends, I am able to function as an independent professional woman as a registered nurse, caring for and helping my patients. That is what I have always wanted to do, yet I always wanted to have three or four children to love and care for as well."

Now lying in bed next to me, with a smile on her face, she would say, "give me a kiss, man. In my capacity as a mother and as a professional nurse, I know at the end of the day, regardless, I always have you, my dear husband who loves me." We snuggled closer together as we fell asleep.

CHAPTER 27

The Schumacher Family

I RECALL THE FIRST TIME MARY and I became aware of the Schumacher family. We had just purchased our house, and we went to check it out a final time before moving in. Mary was standing in the living room, looking out the front window, when she first saw Mrs. Anne Schumacher.

I am not sure what would pique her interest, but Mary called, with a humorous tone, "Willis, come here, babe!" I was intrigued by the tone of Mary's voice. I quickly stood by her side in the living room, looking out the front window.

Mary said, "after we came into the house, the lady across the street walked to the neighbor's house (the Hicks) next door, and it caught my attention. Willis, I am curious, observing the way she went to the house as if they were gathering to scrutinize us as an African-American family. I wonder if that would be her reaction if it were another white family moving into this house.

It didn't take long for that rhetorical question to be answered. After we moved into our house, the Schumacher family welcomed us to the neighborhood. Their kids, Mary, and Ronnie Schumacher, that were the same ages as Willis Jr. and Monica, came over and introduced themselves to our kids. I don't recall if Anne Schumacher and her husband Gene came as a couple or if they came individually and introduced themselves and welcomed us to the community.

The interesting and also encouraging thing was that we received a very friendly welcome from our neighbors. Even more so, our neighbors living in the cluster of six homes in our immediate neighborhood came and introduced themselves to our family in a friendly way.

The parents of the kids' our children ages that Willis Jr. and Monica played with were cordial and decent people. The families that lived closest to our house in the 1300 block of Mullanphy Lane were the Schumacher's and Hicks.' Mary and I established an acquaintance and were neighborly with those two families, although our personal interactions were limited on a social level.

However, within two months, the Henderson's' house was on the right (north) of the Schumacher's house. Mr. and Mrs. Henderson was an African-American family, and they moved into the neighborhood after the Chin family, a Chinese-American family had moved into the neighborhood a month after we moved into the area. The Henderson's (Bobbi and Carl) had one daughter, Stephanie, who was a few years younger than our daughter Monica.

The Henderson's were a few years younger than Mary and I. However, trying to get to know one another as neighbors, we socialized on one or two occasions. Carl and Bobbi accepted our invitation and spent a sociable evening at our house on those occasions with their daughter, Stephanie.

Mary Schumacher and Willis Jr. were the same age, and Ronnie Schumacher, Monica, and Patty Chin were the same age. Patty's sister Virginia was two years older than Willis Jr., and Glenn Hicks was four years older than Willis Jr. These kids from the four families living next door and across the street from one another played exceptionally well together. They presented diverse racial and cultural backgrounds among the four families living in the cluster of homes.

They had the normal reactions of any seven, nine, eleven, and thirteen-year-old kids that got ticked off, or upset with a friend, would have. However, ten minutes later, they all were playing together like nothing had happened. I observed carefully the kids interacting together, and it was obvious to me that they had more in common than differences. They enjoyed playing together and being friends.

I believe these kids got along so well because they were just regular kids raised with core Christian and moral values. Glenn and Ronnie, having known each other the longest, in spite of the age difference, were closer friends than either was with Willis Jr. Regardless, all three of the boys had a good friendship and had fun playing together.

Mary Schumacher was two years older than Monica, and Mary had a bossy personality. Monica was also used to having her way, and I spoiled her to a degree. Therefore, the two girls didn't establish as strong a friendship as the three boys did.

With similar personalities, Mary and Monica would often clash. Neither wanted to give in or compromise on the other's suggestions or interests. Monica wanted to have things go her way, the same as Mary wanted her way. However, Mary and Monica got along well enough that they could coexist and have fun with the other kids. I also believe Mary being two years older than Monica factored into Mary instinctively wanting to be the dominant personality in their friendship.

Monica had a much closer friendship with Patty Chin than with Mary. It was normal when three or four kids do hang out together that two kids in the group would be "tighter with each other" than the third person in their circle. Because Patty and Monica were the same age, I believe that facilitated the relationship between them being closer than individually with Mary Schumacher.

Mrs. Chin had passed (died) before the Chin family moved to Florissant. Mr. Chin owned a Chinese restaurant in St. Louis, city, and during the weekdays, he stayed in the city and came home on Mondays after the weekend. The Chin family had an adult housekeeper, Lillian, who lived at their home and looked after the children.

Raymond was the only son and the oldest child. He was 16 years old, Virginia was 11, Patty was seven, and Christy, the family's youngest, was four. Lillian eventually stopped working for the Chin family; Raymond took the responsibility, in his father's absence, of managing the household as a teenager.

Mary (Drake) became sort of a surrogate mother-figure for their family as Raymond would discuss female issues involving the girls, as Virginia became a teenager, and Patty was getting older. Mary would marvel at the responsibility Raymond had undertaken for his young sisters. He would periodically come to our house and talk with Mary when the situation of having that tremendous family responsibility seemed to overwhelm him.

At times as a 17-year-old kid, he was shouldering a heavy responsibility; and Mary helped him in any way she could. When Raymond was inundated with issues he had no experience handling, Mary was always available to counsel and help him navigate the issues.

Because of Monica's friendship with Patty, our family had a special connection with the Chin family. During our Christmas vacation in December 1973, Patty traveled with us to Los Angeles, California, to visit my brother Charles Drake and his family.

Mary sometimes talked with Virginia directly, as she was becoming a young teenager. Raymond, with the responsibility he was shouldering, did well in high school. I believe he graduated high school in June 1974. Subsequent to our family moving from Florissant, MO., we only had intermittent communications with the Chin family.

With interactions with the Schumacher's, we learned they had moved to Florissant, MO., in 1966 from O'Neill, Nebraska, a small town, and they had only lived in Florissant three years. Gene Schumacher periodically talked about wanting to move back to his home state of Nebraska.

Mary and I were aware of the polarized and sometimes hostile climate in the predominantly white St. Louis County communities as African-American families moved into the neighborhoods. We moved into our house on May 30, 1969. I am convinced the primary reason we didn't experience any ugly racial incidents when we moved to Florissant was that we had bought a house that we were spiritually guided to purchase.

Notwithstanding the fact that Mary and I were both reasonably informed and intelligent, our children were reasonably bright, with good home training and proper upbringing. I also think that having access to resources, we were able to sufficiently maintain our house in proper repair, the same as, or more so, than any of our neighbors could demonstrate. We were as capable as anyone, regardless of ethnicity or race, of living in this community.

All these factors helped to eliminate potential racial conflict or incidents. The neighbors, in truth, didn't have the "stereotypical" images or situations they could cast on me, Mary, or our kids, because it would be false.

The Schumacher's had seven children ranging in age from seventeen or eighteen years old down to their youngest son Tommy, who was born in December 1968. He was one month shy of being 2 years older than our son Kermit Matthew, who was born in November 1970.

Coincidentally, that meant there was a child in our family close to or the same age as a child in the Schumacher family. Tommy and Kermit did not get to play together or get to know one another well. Not like Mary, Ronnie, Willis, and Monica did during the five years we were neighbors.

Mary and Ronnie attended St. Sabrina Catholic Elementary School, located at 1625 Swallow Lane in Florissant, but the older kids attended the Hazelwood District Public Junior High and High Schools.

My wife, Mary, and I did not socialize with the parents of the kids that Willis Jr. and Monica played with. We were always neighborly and would have cordial conversations, particularly outside in our front yards. Mary and I both personally thought well of Gene and Anne Schumacher. They were good people and neighbors.

It was only once or twice that either Gene and Anne or Mary and I had visited each other's homes as a couple. Mary and I were not the type of people that visited the home of our neighbors. When we lived in St. Louis City, we didn't visit our neighbors' homes.

Gene and I often stood in our front yard having a conversation, talking across the street to one another. One day Gene and I were talking, and he told me he worked for the federal government at the FAA (Federal Aviation Administration) located at Lambert St. Louis Airport, and he was a GS-12 Supply Cataloger.

We laughed politely as I told Gene I also work for the federal government at MECOM (Mobility Equipment Command), the Army Logistic Agency located at 4300 Goodfellow Boulevard, and I was a GS-9 Supply Cataloger. It was interesting that Gene and I had several things in common, including our job classification.

Gene, Anne, and their children helped make living in Florissant a normal and enjoyable experience for our family, particularly for our children. Mary and Ronnie Schumacher, along with the Chin family and Glen Hicks, were Willis Jr. and Monica's best friends in the neighborhood. Stephanie Henderson was younger and only played sparingly with the older children in the circle of five families in the cluster of houses.

Instead of Gene and I talking from across the street, as we often did, I went over to Gene's front yard one day. We were talking, and with a slight hesitation, Gene said, "Willis, I remember when your family moved into your house. I said to Anne, oh well, here goes the neighborhood." I listen intently, with truth being spoken by a neighbor that had the typical reaction when an African-American family moved into their neighborhood.

Then he said, "Willis, you have been the best neighbor I could ever imagine having. In fact, my wife Anne constantly uses you as an example when she tells me what I should be doing around my house. Her comment was, "look at Mr. Drake, he keeps his lawn always looking good, and he does this, and he does that, around his house, etc."

Gene was smiling sheepishly as he said, "Willis, man, you are a hard act to follow." Gene and I just laughed as two neighbors just talking small talk as men, being honest about his initial erroneous perception about my family because we are African-American.

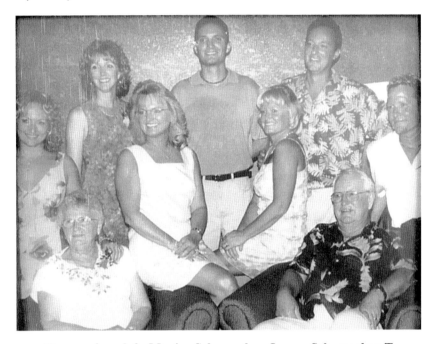

Top row from left: Monica Schumacher, Jeanne Schumacher, T ommy Schumacher, Ronnie Schumacher, Ricky Schumacher. Bottom row from left: (Mrs.) Anne Schumacher, Julie Schumacher, Mary Schumacher and (Mr.) Gene Schumacher.

Our family lived in our home at 1340 Mullanphy Lane, Florissant, Mo, for five years. On June 6, 1974, the Schumacher's moved from Florissant to North Platte, Nebraska, to live. Within a few months, after the Schumacher's had moved, in late August during the summer of 1974, I relocated our family from Florissant to Springfield, Michigan, to live. It is a small city located five miles outside Battle Creek, Michigan.

We were moving away from our combined, structured, very close Drake and Byas families. We were collectively one family, which centered on Mary's family living in East St. Louis; and my family living in St. Louis. It was a very emotional time for our entire family moving from Florissant. Willis Jr. and Monica were basically teenagers, and our moving to Michigan had the greatest impact on them.

However, as we settled into our new home, the kids made new friends and adjusted to the new Springfield, Michigan community. Willis Jr., more so than Monica, stayed in touch with Mary and Ronnie Schumacher for a brief time after they had moved.

Mary always planned our summer vacations, and we traveled using the northern route to California for our 1975 summer vacation. Mary wanted to visit the Air Force Academy on the trip. We had always traveled the southern route to California and had seen the Grand Canyon, the Petrified Forest, and other landmarks of interest traveling that route.

Knowing that we would travel through Nebraska, we contacted Gene and Anne Schumacher to let them know we would be passing through Nebraska on our July vacation trip, and if convenient, we would stop and say hello to them.

As time drew near, we made our travel plans so we would arrive in North Platte, Nebraska, in the afternoon. Like clockwork, it was 12:30 pm when we arrived at the Schumacher's home. Our intentions were to stop, say hello, and visit for an hour. However, Gene and Anne insisted that our family stay the night at their house, and we did.

It was gratifying to see the Schumacher family again, and the kids were excited and reconnected like they were in Florissant again. Gene, Anne, Mary, and I got caught up on how our families were doing. Mary and Anne talked about the trials of being a parent of young teenagers. Anne assured Mary, this is my second time, so with Mary and Ronnie, I know how to handle it. Just hang in there, Mary; it will be okay.

As we laughed, talked, and socialized, collectively, we agreed that the kids had adjusted well to the new area where they now live. They had settled into the school system and had made a social circle of new friends. As we continued talking, it was now evening time, and we ordered pizza for dinner; the kids huddled together, consuming their pizza and reminiscing.

As we ate dinner, we had a fluid conversation, and Mary and I learned that Gene and Anne both felt comfortable living back in their home state of Nebraska. Gene still worked for the FAA and was able to transfer to a job in North Platte, Nebraska. "Several years later, talking with Anne Schumacher, she told me that when they moved to North Platte." Gene's new job with the FAA was as an Electronics Engineer classification. He was the manager of all of Nebraska's transmitting sites for airplane flights in the area. He would say, "I enjoy the job, but I hate all the paperwork."

We also learned that Anne came from a large family, and she was the 10th of fourteen children. She also came from a family with a history of long longevity, and her mother lived to be 110 years old.

It was close to 9:00 o'clock when we got ready for bed. Anne showed us to the room where we would sleep; and said, "I hope you will be comfortable sleeping tonight; good night, and we will see you in the morning."

As families do, the girls (Mary and Monica Schumacher) made accommodations in their bedroom for Monica; and Ronnie and Tommy huddled up in their bedroom where Willis Jr. and Kermit slept.

We woke up early the following day after a restful night's sleep and got ready to hit the highway. We thanked Gene and Anne for their gracious hospitality, and the kids lingered a minute, saying their goodbyes to the Schumacher kids. It was close to 7:30 am when we bid farewell to the Schumacher's and headed to the highway.

It was a short but very enjoyable visit. Staying at the Schumacher's home and sharing time with their family again is still a memorable experience for me. Through social media, the kids (Willis Jr. and Ronnie) are in touch periodically with one another.

Anne Schumacher sent me a letter with her family background information and information about Gene's job in North Platte. I have sent her a birthday card several times for her birthday, and Anne Schumacher celebrated her 90th birthday on December 30, 2022.

CHAPTER 28

―――――― ◇ ――――――

Reemployment With The
Federal Government

―――――― ◇ ――――――

F OR OUR FUTURE LONG-TERM FAMILY security, Mary and I agreed that I should pursue employment with the federal government as opposed to staying employed in the private sector. We both understood returning to federal civil service employment would require us to relocate to another state. I submitted job applications to three government agencies in Rock Island, Illinois, Des Moines, Iowa, and Battle Creek, Michigan.

Now in retrospect, I smile with internal joy when I recall Mary's comment when she said with such conviction, and the confidence and determination she displayed just magnified her words. "Willis, baby, I will go wherever a job takes you! As long as we are together, that's all that matters to me. Moving will not be a big problem for the kids either at their ages."

Surprisingly, within a few months, I received a job offer from two of the three agencies that I had applied. Shortly after that, I had a telephone interview with the branch chief, Ms. Johno Gailey, of the North Atlantic Treaty Organization (NATO), located at the Defense Logistics Services Center (DLSC) in Battle Creek, Michigan. I accepted the GS-9 Supply Cataloger position in the NATO branch.

It had been a year since I was last in Battle Creek when I worked for the McDonnell Douglas Aircraft Corporation. That was when I had the spiritual revelation clearly informing me, "You are going to live here soon." Now I was on the threshold of moving my family to live in the Battle Creek (Springfield) area.

During our dinner conversations, we informed the kids that we would be moving from the Florissant (St. Louis) area. We often reinforced that Battle Creek was only an eight-hour drive from St. Louis. Therefore, it's not that far away, and you can visit your grandparents and cousins often.

The school year had ended, and it was now the middle of summer. Willis Jr. and Monica were participating in their Florissant summer sports league for the fourth year. They both were arguably the best players on their baseball and softball teams, respectively.

Playing the ball games seemed to minimize their focus on moving soon. In July, both of their teams played in the league championship play-offs. When their season ended, their teams had a farewell celebration for them.

I had to report to Battle Creek in mid-July to start my new job. Without blinking her eye, in my absence, Mary would make the necessary adjustments for her and the kids during this time of transition. Mary would function as a single mother for seven weeks, shouldering the responsibility for our family until I could relocate the family to the Battle Creek/ Springfield areas.

I felt somewhat guilty leaving Mary to pack up our household, and manage the kids' daily activities, while I was in Battle Creek working. This was just another example of the strong woman that she was. She would do whatever was necessary to support and care for our family.

Mary was a pillar of strength leading up to my leaving for Battle Creek. She was a stalwart every day in front of the children. However, in our solitude, Mary expressed reservations concerning my being away for seven weeks.

She expressed how much she depended on me and the strength I gave her just knowing I was there in the house. Then that smile would appear on her face, and she would say, "I know these weeks will fly by." I would hug her and let her know we are blessed together and she and the kids will be fine during my short absence.

Saturday morning, just before 7:00 am, I had my lingering emotional embrace with Mary and the kids. I knew it would be seven weeks before I could embrace her like this again. I wanted to savor this personal moment with Mary and remember this feeling during the seven weeks I would be alone in Battle Creek.

When I was walking out the front door, I knew it would take approximately eight hours to drive the 435 miles to Battle Creek. However, I made exceptional time traveling, and it was close to 3:00 pm when I arrived at the hotel in the Lakeview Township, five miles outside of Battle Creek, Michigan.

I immediately called Mary to let her know I had arrived safely in Battle Creek. Mary was surprised when she answered the phone, that I had arrived in Battle Creek already. We talked for a few minutes, and I spoke to the kids, also.

During the next seven weeks, for the first time, our family would have to endure being separated. However, Mary and I had five years of experience to draw on emotionally, from being separated when she was in nursing school and living on campus during the weekdays. The same as it was then, together, Mary and I could endure anything!

Battle Creek Housing
I knew Mary could not make a house-hunting trip, so my first priority was finding a house for our family. Cecil Black and his wife Gerri, good friends from St. Louis, had arranged for their real estate agent, Virginia, to show me houses in the surrounding Battle Creek area.

I arrived for work Monday morning at the Battle Creek Federal Center (BCFC) with the normal uncertainties of any first day on the job. I was surprised that two former coworkers from St. Louis, James Poe, and Rudolf (Rudy) Kuesters, were also my coworkers in the NATO cataloging branch.

After work, that first day, Virginia, the real estate agent, showed me several really nice houses for sale throughout the surrounding Battle Creek township areas. However, I was reluctant to buy a house without Mary seeing it first. Together, we always had input on any major decision that impacted our lives. Therefore, I didn't want to decide independently on purchasing a house without Mary's input.

After a month, I still had not found a house for our family. During a morning break, Rudy Kuesters mentioned his family lived in the Fort Custer Housing Complex, located in Springfield, Michigan, a few miles West of Battle Creek.

Every night When Mary and I talked, we discussed the possibility of temporarily renting an apartment. Mary stressed if we had to live in an apartment temporarily, she wanted four bedrooms, a living room, a kitchen, and a dining room. She also emphasized she wanted to live in a safe neighborhood.

I looked at two apartments, and they both met Mary's requirements. I signed a month-to-month lease, for an apartment at the Fort Custer Apartment Complex. Therefore, when we are ready to buy a house, I could terminate the apartment lease with a thirty-day notice.

I also prompted Mary to prepare the kids that living at the Fort Custer Apartment Complex would be vastly different than living in our house in Florissant, MO., which was in an upscale middle-income community. The apartment complex was safe, clean, and respectable, but it was not the same housing standard that Mary and the kids were familiar with, living in our Florissant home.

The city of Springfield, Michigan, had its own school system, City Hall, Police and Fire Departments, and the administrative support that an independent city required. The population was approximately 3,000 people compared to Battle Creek's approximately thirty-five (35,000) thousand people. Overall, our new community of Battle Creek & Springfield, Michigan was a small town, compared to the broad St. Louis metropolitan area, with a population over a million people.

Returning Home to Get the Family
However, I still remember vividly that Thursday evening phone call from Mary, the day before I returned home. She sounded so distraught, and she was sobbing dreadfully. I was startled, hearing Mary crying with such intensity. With a sense of urgency, I asked her what was wrong.

As she regained her composure, in between her tears, she conveyed the events that had happened. Recounting, the entire week had gone haywire. She spewed out the two horrific episodes of what had happened during the week.

She told me she had a "Slumber Party" for Monica and her girl cousins, Paulette Tolden (who periodically spent weekends with Monica), Shappell Cody, Crystal Sykes, and Antoria Harris, to enjoy the week together.

The girls were playing on the patio, and Paulette cut her big toe, and instantly her right foot was covered with blood. The kids ran into the house, and Shappell was crying, screaming that Paulette had cut off her big toe. I cleaned up the cut on Paulette's foot, put a bandage on the cut, and stopped the bleeding. We rushed to the hospital's Emergency Room (ER)

I am not sure if the admitting Registered Nurse (RN) just wasn't familiar with admitting African-Americans for treatment at this hospital's ER. She displayed a rude and unprofessional attitude.

After we had checked in with the admitting nurse, Paulette sat in the registration area for too long without a doctor seeing her injured foot.

Willis, I did not go "crazy" on that nurse, but first, I injected my hard-earned professional qualifications as an RN, trained and educated at Homer G. School of nursing, one of the best nursing schools in the country.

I dressed her down in a manner she will never forget. I let that uncooperative nurse and her supervisor, who had now appeared, know that if they did not treat my young cousin immediately, they would have the biggest lawsuit on their hands, and I would have their jobs too. "Willis, it was amazing the speed at which Paulette was treated. Thank goodness, medically, her cut was superficial, in spite of all the blood from Paulette's foot initially."

As Mary continued talking, the situation with the neighbor whose backyard was adjacent to ours that lived on Aspen Lane became concerning. Their teenage son, who was several years older than Willis Jr., perpetrated a verbal racist-laced assault and physical threats against Birdie.

Mary said, "Willis, during the five years we lived in our house, there was no meaningful communication between our families. I know the only reason that incident happened was because that stupid teenager knew you were out of town." If you were here, that coward would have stayed in his racist cocoon!

I reminded Mary that I would be home in less than 24 hours tomorrow evening. Just remember that we were blessed despite the incidents of the week, and everything will be okay. I also talked with Willis Jr. and told him to watch out and protect himself; and continue looking out for his mom, sister, and little brother; I would see him tomorrow evening.

I let Mary know that our family would be protected in my absence. As we hung up the telephone, I felt certain we would both sleep well tonight, anticipating seeing one another tomorrow evening.

On Friday evening, August 23rd, I had my air flight reservations confirmed, and I was excited to relocate my family to our new home in the Springfield/Battle Creek area. I was super hyped with anticipation of seeing my family.

CHAPTER 29

Going Home to Get My Family

I WAS ABLE TO SLEEP VERY well Thursday night; I woke up Friday morning full of energy. In the shower, I was singing our favorite song, "My Girl." I got dressed super-fast. My suitcase was packed, and I had settled my hotel bill last night. I checked out of the hotel and left to go to work. I had a special hop-in-my-step.

At work the entire day, my mind was focused on going home, and I repeatedly glanced at the clock. Finally, it was four o'clock, and I rushed from the Federal Center to my Fort Custer Apartment Complex, where our family would be living.

The apartment was ten minutes from the Battle Creek Kellogg Airport, and my friend Cecil Black dropped me off at the airport. In the airport terminal, I heard the final announcement echoing throughout the lobby for all passengers to check in and board the airplane going to Chicago.

In short order, the airplane was loaded, roared down the runway, and took off at 5:00 pm. The wheels lifted, and within minutes I was airborne. As the plane gained a higher altitude, Battle Creek became invisible. Then I relaxed in my seat as the flight to O'Hare Chicago Airport would arrive at six o'clock CST.

The flight had taken less than an hour when it landed in Chicago—exiting the plane, I had to maneuver through the crowd to make my connecting flight to St. Louis. I boarded the large jet aircraft and got seated. My thoughts intensified, knowing I would be able to see the kids and embrace Mary in a little over an hour.

The flight landed at 6:30 pm on schedule, and I proceeded to the passenger pickup area, where I immediately saw my big sister Shirley. We greeted one another enthusiastically, and we exited the airport immediately. Driving home, Shirley filled me in on what was happening in the Florissant neighborhood. She lived at 2384 Stoney End Court, in Florissant, fifteen minutes from my house.

I knew we would arrive at my home in twenty-five minutes. Shirley pulled into the driveway, and I went into the house, and Mary was standing in the living room. She said, hi, babe, with a big smile on her face, coming toward me. Before she could reach me, Kermit rushed reaching for me to pick him up.

I swooped him up in the air, and Monica came and hugged me. There was laughter and joy going around. I felt so good being able to hug my kids, particularly my daughter Monica. Willis Jr. was a teenager, and we shook hands like "men."

At four years old, Kermit reigned supreme as the baby in the family. Mary walked to me, and we embraced and kissed. Kermit was hugging my neck, and he wanted to be my primary focus. My niece "Little Shirley" (Shirley Drake-Hairston) extracted Kermit from my arms so I could embrace Mary more affectionately for a moment.

Tenderly we just embraced in silence as we had a polite kiss. I know the emotional part of our family moving to the Springfield/Battle Creek area would impact our entire family living in St. Louis and East St. Louis.

During the week, family members helped Mary get situated for the move to Battle Creek. My dad assisted with renting the U-Haul truck. Then on Friday, he supervised my nephews, Wayne Gooch, and Stephan

Cody, along with Willis Jr. and Mary's brother David Byas, on how to pack our furniture securely in the truck. The only item Mary didn't pack was the mattress for our bed.

We had prepped the kids, the best we could, for moving away from our family. Having to separate from their grandparents; and their cousins, whom they had grown up with since they were babies, would not be easy.

"The cousins" living in St. Louis were remarkably close growing up. Notably, Little Shirley, Wayne Gooch, Crystal Sykes-Grimmett, Stephone Cody, Shappell Cody-Rice, Sharronda Cody-Boyd, and Shondria (Shon) Cody-Wharton visited their grandparents' home often during the week too. Also, their Harris' cousins, Flarzell, Wakita (Kiki) Harris, DeAndre Harris, Vititia Harris-Peoples, Antoria Harris-Javier, Marco Harris, and Apollos Steven Harris; and their Drake cousins Deborah Drake, Cynthia Drake-Ballwin, and Brenda Drake, Dana Drake; and Charles Drake Jr., Paula Drake-Miller, and Arcola (Queenie) Drake-Aikens.

Mary's cousins, with the exception of Maurice (Sonny) and Alvin Tolden, were younger. Her cousin Paul Tolden was a few years younger, and she was more of a role model for her younger female cousins (Barbara Ann, Linda, Jo-Jo (Ardella), and Renee) living in East St. Louis.

We were in the final stage of moving. The U-Haul rental truck was in the driveway, packed, and ready to leave in the morning. I only had to put our mattress on the truck, and we would be ready to hit the highway.

The Drake cousins spend the night at my sister Shirley's house. Little Shirley spent the night at our house to keep Kermit occupied for the night.

Mary's brother David stayed overnight at our house and would be traveling with us, riding in the car with Mary and helping her drive. I would drive the U-Haul truck, and I had purchased an airline ticket so David could fly back to St. Louis on Sunday.

Kermit was the oldest of the cousins of his mother's siblings in his generation. However, Mary didn't articulate it, but I could tell that moving away from her family, she would miss them, particularly her "little sisters" Mona and Margaret Ann. Mary had said her goodbyes to her parents and siblings when they dropped David off at our house Friday.

It had been seven weeks since I had been home, but it seemed longer to me. Initially, being home that night was a little awkward. Kermit Matthew, not having seen me, his dad, in almost two months, wanted to sleep in the bed with Mary and me.

Somehow, Little Shirley managed to persuade Kermit, her godson, to sleep in his bedroom with her. Therefore, Mary and I were able to have our private time together.

I felt great waking up this morning with Mary lying next to me. She was cradled in my arms, and feeling her warmth against my body, reminded me of what I had missed these past seven weeks. Without Mary saying a word, the smile on her face expressed the joy she also had waking up lying next to me.

Now there was a light tap on our door, and suddenly it opened, and Kermit came into our bedroom, and he jumped on the mattress between Mary and me. "Good morning," as he hugged Mary and me simultaneously. Playfully, I asked, "Did you sleep okay last night? He said with a frown on his face, "Daddy, I wanted to sleep with you and momma last night, but little Shirley was afraid to sleep in my room by herself.

Smiling, I didn't respond to Kermit's comment; I tickled his stomach and said, "come on, you need to get dressed. We must hit the road early to get to our new home in Springfield (Battle Creek), Michigan. Mary told Kermit, "You know that's where we will be living now, right." Unenthusiastically, he responded, yes, mom, I know.

Now with a sense of urgency, she ushered Kermit out of our room, stating, it's 6:30, so please ask little Shirley to help you get dressed." We need to hurry up to hit the road by 8:00 o'clock. Okay, get moving; we are on a tight schedule this morning.

Kermit left the room begrudgingly, saying, "oh, mom." I was laughing to myself as I realized the simple ordinary things I had missed these several weeks that were just routine and elementary but enjoyable.

Mary and I started moving quickly, and she jumped in the shower first. Now it was 7:15, and Kermit, Little Shirley, and David were up and dressed. My sister Shirley, with the nieces and nephews, arrived at the house around 7:20 am. David had Willis Jr., Wayne, and Stephone, help him put the mattress in the U-Haul truck. The Chin girls (Virginia, Patty, and Christy) came to the house to bid our family farewell, and the girls were commiserating with each other as if they would never see one another again.

The doorbell rang, and Monica, with a jubilant voice, said, it's grand momma and granddaddy. She opened the door and hugged her grandmother. Entering the house, my mom hugged Monica and said, "come on now "Miss Renee," and put that pretty smile on your face. I don't want you to be sad, okay."

Mom and dad were now standing in the living room, and Mary and I greeted mother with a hug, and I shook my dad's hand. Immediately, mother ushered Mary into the kitchen to have a private conversation and to say their goodbyes.

As Mary and mother retreated to the kitchen, I thanked my dad for showing the "young nephews" how to tie down the furniture and pack the U-Haul truck securely, so nothing would be damaged when driving the truck.

Dad laughed and said, "they thought just putting the furniture on the truck was all they needed to do. Not realizing while you are driving the truck, furniture could bounce around if it is not tied down." Dad had a big smile on his face that transformed quickly into laughter as we both were now laughing.

Mary and I were blessed to have our families' support now and throughout our marriage, as we did. The U-Haul rental truck was basically packed and ready to go when I arrived home Friday evening.

My dad had cautioned me to drive safely and not be in a rush getting to Battle Creek. As I was pulling out of the driveway, I looked at my dad through the truck's windshield, and as I had known all my life, particularly during my married life, my dad was proud of my family and me.

My mother had bided us farewell earlier when we were inside the house. She told Mary and me, "You'll have a blessed life in your new home in Springfield, Michigan. Then she said, Willis, continue to stay as you are, and you and Mary always depend on each other." As was her normal practice, mother didn't come outside the house when we were leaving.

Our neighbors were standing in front of our house, and Monica's friend Patty Chin was crying emotionally. It was good to see the love and farewell blessings, but it was also emotional, as our family members and neighbors were outside our house to say bye.

Monica and Patty were best friends, and we had taken Patty with us on our Christmas vacation to Los Angeles, California, the previous Christmas. Like so many young girls, Patty was awestruck by Michael Jackson and the Jackson five music group, and she got to see them at the Rose Bowl Parade in Pasadena, California, on January 1, 1974.

We were moving from Florissant, but we still owned our house. We had rented the house to a young married couple with one preschool-age child. We thought they would be excellent tenants and would take care of the property. My sister Shirley Drake-Sykes was the property manager to address any maintenance issues, and she received the monthly rent payments to deposit in the account I had set up.

Sitting in the driver's seat of our car, Mary was composed as she pulled away from the house. Mary's brother, David, Monica, and Kermit Matthew were in the car with her. Driving a long distance on the highway would be a new experience for Mary.

Willis Jr. was in the truck with me, and our plan was to follow behind Mary's car, traveling in the highway's right lane as much as possible.

It was Willis Jr.'s job to ensure he could always see his mother's car in front of us.

We drove Interstate Highway I-55/I-57 to Interstate I-94 on our way to Springfield, Michigan. We had planned stops outside Chicago, and as needed, we stopped to eat and gas up along the trip. Mary and I travel at a consistent speed of 65 to 70 miles an hour.

I discovered later that the rental truck had a governor devise on the gas accelerator, and the speed would only accelerate to seventy miles an hour, which worked fine for me. Mary and I both were comfortable driving at that speed.

During our rest and meal stops, Mary nurtured her young daughter Monica, who was experiencing an emotional situation moving away from her friends and family members. I watched Mary walking to the rest area with her arms around Monica's waist as she tried to cheer her up.

I was fascinated by observing Mary and her motherly touch, which was so comforting for Monica. I marveled at Mary's compassion and maternal instincts towards her near-teenage daughter Monica.

Willis Jr., especially Monica, started to cheer up as we got farther away from St. Louis. Now at the rest stops, conversations, laughter, and chatter continued in the car and truck. The kids were gesturing with hand signals back and forth between the vehicles. Within an hour of our destination, our whole family was looking forward to arriving in Springfield, MI., to start our lives anew.

I had told the kids that we would be twenty minutes from Springfield when we got to Kalamazoo, Michigan. Seeing the Kalamazoo highway sign, I beeped the horn, and Monica looked out the back car window, motioning to Willis Jr. that the sign had Kalamazoo exit. I could see the grins on their faces as they waved to one another.

Twenty-five minutes later, we arrived at the Fort Custer Apartment Complex. I backed the truck into our assigned parking space, and everybody got out of the vehicles. I hugged Mary and told her she did a fantastic job driving the highway. Monica laughed and said, daddy, I know momma can drive on the highway. Everyone was in a jovial mood and was thankful that we had a safe trip driving to our new home.

With my Bible in hand, we entered our apartment, formed a circle holding hands, and I read the 23rd Psalm. I prayed that our family would have a blessed life in our new Springfield, Michigan home, the same as we had in Florissant.

Now, Mary's attention was focused on the aesthetic of the apartment. Inconspicuously, I was observing Mary's facial expression and body language as she walked through the living room, dining room, and kitchen areas; she was visually and thoroughly inspecting the first-floor level of the apartment.

She put her arm around Monica's shoulders and said let's go upstairs and check out the bedrooms. A few minutes later, they returned downstairs, and Mary was smiling. She commented that all the rooms are large, and I like the hardwood floors throughout the apartment. Monica, smiling, also agreed with her mother.

Mary always accentuated the positive aspects of everything, and she appeared pleased with the apartment. But more than anything, having our family together was most important. Overall, Willis Jr. and Monica seemed pleased, and Kermit Matthew went with the flow of his big brother and sister.

Mary had completed her initial perusal of the apartment when our friends, Cecil and Gerri Black, arrived with their three-year-old son, Kenny. Cecil came to help unload the truck, and Gerri helped Mary and Monica arrange the small items inside the apartment.

David, Willis Jr., Cecil, and I unloaded the truck; it was more fun than work. Mary and Gerri were laughing, cautioning Cecil and me not to have a heart attack, trying to outdo David and Birdie unloading the truck.

Mission Accomplished

We finished unloading the truck before it turned dark that evening, and I returned the U-Haul truck to the rental company on East Michigan Avenue.

I returned to the apartment, and Mary said, "Willis, everybody is hungry, and we want to have pizza." With his dry humor, David asked if they served beer with the pizza. With a big grin, Cecil chimed in; David, that's how I like my pizza, man, with a beer. They slapped their hands and decided we were going to "Pizza Hut" to eat.

The Pizza Hut was at Capital and Columbia avenues, and it will take about 15 minutes to drive there from your apartment. We agreed to freshen up first and meet at Pizza Hut in an hour.

It was ironic that the first evening with my family in Springfield, Michigan, we were in the Pizza Hut, eating pizza with Cecil and Gerri Black, our only friends in the area. We reminisced about knowing one another for over a dozen years, dating back to 1963 when we worked together at the Mart Building in downtown St. Louis.

Leaving Pizza Hut, Gerri and Mary hugged, and she reminded Mary, "I will have Virginia, the real estate agent, call you in a couple of weeks. She can help you find the right house to buy in this area. Mary said, "be sure to give Virginia my contact information. I will be looking to find a house as soon as possible." We left the parking lot heading home.

Mary wanted David to eat breakfast before leaving for the airport. So on the way home, we stopped at the Kroger grocery store and bought food for breakfast. We also drove past the Battle Creek Kellogg's Airport. Mary said, "Willis, is that the airport?" Yes, baby, as I slowed down so everyone could see the small airport. Yep, that's the airport I flew out of Friday going home.

David said, "Will (which he called me, short for Willis), I hope the big jet airplanes fly from this small airport." In a serious voice, "sorry, David, only the small propeller engine airplanes fly out of this airport, and they only carry about twenty passengers."

"Will, what time do I need to be at the airport? My flight leaves at 8:45 in the morning." Hey, it will only take ten minutes to drive to the airport, and I will get you there at 8:00 am.

We entered the apartment, and Mary said, "okay, everyone is tired, so why don't we all go to bed? David said, "Pookie, I am ready to hit the sack, and I can hear the bed calling my name." The kids laughed at their uncle David's comment.

I put my arms around Mary's shoulders as we headed upstairs. At that moment, my thoughts were simple, after seven weeks, our family would now spend the night together under the same roof, and I knew everything would be all right going forward here in Springfield, Michigan.

I woke up the next morning feeling terrific with Mary by my side and my family together, safe, and secure under the same roof with me. It felt awesome. I sat up in bed and gazed down, looking at Mary, who was in a deep sleep. I was feeling a little mischievous.

First, I called her name very softly, and she barely stirred. I then leaned down and softly blew in her ear. That normally always generated a slight smile on her face, and she started to stir, but she was not quite awake yet.

I blew in her ear again softly, and her smile broadened, and she said, "Willis is that you trying to wake me up?" She opened her eyes, and I could only smile. I was thinking about these trivial things I had missed for seven weeks. Now I was getting back to our normal life with Mary in bed by my side.

Now laughing, she said, "man, I know I asked you to wake me up, but you haven't changed. You just can't stand to see me sleeping when you are awake, can you?" My soft laugh changed into a roar, and I kissed Mary as she stretched her arms up in the air and wrapped them around my neck.

Okay baby "watch out now, David has an early flight this morning, and you don't want him to miss his plane, do you?" We both laughed as we rose to get out of bed. It was still early, only 6:45 in the morning. We got dressed quickly, and then Mary tapped on the bedroom door where David was sleeping and asked if he was awake. His response was immediate, as he opened the door and said good morning, Pookie; I have been awake for a while now, sis.

Okay, come downstairs and eat your breakfast before you leave for the airport. In her big sister's role, she was fixing eggs, bacon, toast, and apple juice for David's breakfast, cautioning him that it would be sometime this evening before he arrived home.

David ate a heartily breakfast at the dining room table, and I sat at the table with him, but I did not eat breakfast. We talked, and he was very anxious about flying. I tried to alleviate his concern about flying on his maiden airplane flight. The kids came downstairs, said their goodbyes, gave hugs and handshakes and thanked their uncle David for helping us move.

Mary hugged David, and they exchanged their big sister and little brother's personal comments. David and I drove from the apartment building, with Mary standing and waving goodbye to her brother.

David was still nervous, notwithstanding our earlier conversation, regarding this would be his first time flying on an airplane. At the airport, I parked the car and went inside the airport terminal with David. We had waited 15 minutes when we heard the announcement that David's flight was now boarding.

David was also my "young brother," the same as he was Mary's. We shook hands and man-hugged; I told him to just relax and that he would have a good flight. As he walked towards the airplane, I reminded him to call us when he got home. He turned and looked at me, said okay, Will, and boarded the plane.

David's flight itinerary was from Battle Creek to Chicago, with a connecting flight from Chicago to St. Louis. I stood in the airport terminal to ensure David's flight departed on schedule. It was as if I was over-seeing my "little brother" flying home, who had helped me immensely to relocate my family over 400 miles away from our previous home. I was confident that David's air flight from Chicago to St. Louis would be more comfortable for him, flying on the larger jet airplane.

--- ◇ ---

CHAPTER 30

Springfield and Battle Creek, Michigan

--- ◇ ---

MARY WAS IN THE LIVING room sitting on the couch when I entered the house. Like a big sister, she wanted to know if David's flight got off okay. I sat down next to her, laughing. I confirmed that David's plane left on time, but he was still a little nervous about flying.

I asked Mary, "Did the kids go back to bed? I know they had a long hard day's work yesterday, but we still have much to get done today. Mary, now facing me and smiling, said, "Willis, let the kids sleep; they earned it."

Anyway, I need some isolation time to plan how I want to decorate this apartment. It has a natural aesthetic appearance. Observing Mary, I could tell her imagination was in full gear and in short order; the apartment would look and feel like our home.

Later that morning, the kids came downstairs, and Willis Jr., with his chest protruding somewhat, announced, "Uncle David and I did a big job helping to unload the truck. Hey dad, you might want to throw a few extra ducats (dollars) my way." Monica said, "Birdie, don't forget I helped too, and I am not asking for an increase in my allowance. You should be glad that you were able to help us get moved.

Mary intervened to prevent the sibling's verbal jostling, comparing who had helped the most. She said both of you were extremely helpful, and don't forget our little man Kermit chipped in too. We laughed, sitting at the dining room table as a family in our apartment.

In our first family discussion, everyone stated their opinion openly concerning our living arrangement at our Fort Custer apartment. I re-iterated that living in this apartment was temporary and we would buy our own house as soon as your mother and I found a house we would like to buy.

Birdie said, "mom and dad, I think this apartment is fine. We have our own large bedroom, there is space in the basement to store things, and the apartment complex overall seems okay. I saw a few kids my age yesterday, and I am sure I will make friends okay. Monica also agreed that the apartment would be fine until we got our own house.

Mary was optimistic, stating, "Willis, I can learn about different communities to live in, and I will work with a realtor to show me houses in the area." Mary knew when I promised her I would do something, if humanly possible; I would keep my word to her!

Everyone was feeling good about the apartment, and we started taking boxes upstairs to the rooms where they belonged. We were working diligently, and everything was falling into place nicely. The phone rang, Mary answered the phone, and her voice increased an octave, saying, "hi David, you made it home already?" It was 1:45 pm.

Mary walked into the Livingroom and sat on the couch next to me. I could hear David say, "yes, Pookie, I got home about 15 minutes ago." Then Mary put the phone closer between us, and I heard David's muf-fled laugh, and he said, "Pookie, I survived this time; but I don't plan to fly anytime again soon."

Mary handed me the phone. "David, I understand your maiden flight was rough, brother. He responded, "Will, that flight from Battle Creek to Chicago was frightening. I was scared to death flying over Lake

Michigan, and the plane was bouncing up and down in the air. I was saying my prayers, and I thought the plane was going to crash.

With a little levity in his voice, he said, "Will, I was hesitant to get on my connecting flight home. However, flying on a big airplane from Chicago to St. Louis was okay." I returned the phone to Mary, and she said goodbye to David.

Mary and I made phone calls to family and friends, giving them our phone number and mailing address. I had to work the next day, so I said good night early and went upstairs to go to bed.

My daily routine was already established over the past seven weeks, and going to work each morning living in the Battle Creek area was normal now. So I would now get up, trying not to disturb Mary.

It was nearing the start of the school year, and Mary would get the kids registered for school on Monday. Over the next several weeks, Mary finished adding her individualized touch to the apartment; and it started to feel like a home to us that we were used to living in.

Additionally, the first adjustment our family had to make was to a different climate. During August, it was not extremely hot compared to St. Louis. However, during the fall months, starting in late September and early October, the weather was much colder in the Battle Creek area than in the St. Louis area.

On a personal level, Willis Jr. and Monica made new friends living in the apartment complex. Also, the racial demographics in Springfield, Michigan, were similar to Florissant, where Willis Jr. and Monica were one of the three or four African-American children in their school system. Now, in Springfield, Michigan, they probably were one of the five or six African-American children in their Springfield Middle School and Junior High School.

In the Springfield School District, children that turned five years old during the calendar year had to register and attend kindergarten that year. Therefore, Kermit Matthew attended kindergarten from 8:00 am until 12:00 noon starting in September 1974.

However, their school and the total environment of the Springfield and Battle Creek communities were different culturally from St. Louis/ Florissant areas. Comparatively speaking, they were somewhat "small town-ish," more so than St. Louis and Florissant areas, but it was equally racially biased.

During the first several weeks after we moved to Springfield, we visited Mount Zion Methodist Episcopal Church, located at 364 W. Van Buren Street, Battle Creek, MI 49037, and Second Missionary Baptist Church, located at 485 Washington Avenue, Battle Creek, MI 49037. Our family attended Mount Zion Methodist Episcopal Church as our permanent church home.

James (Jim) Wright was a supervisor in the NATO Cataloging Electronic Branch, where I worked. He had a son, James (Jimmy) Wright Jr., who was a year older than Willis Jr., and a daughter Denise Wright (Carethers), who was a year younger than Monica. Shortly after we moved to the Springfield area, Jim invited our family to their home to meet his wife Mildred and their two children. They lived at 62 Hickory Nut Lane, an "exclusive" (upscale) neighborhood in Springfield, Michigan. Their home was ten minutes from Fort Custer.

Mildred and Jim were ten or twelve years older than Mary and I. We needed to establish a meaningful relationship with African-American families living in the surrounding Springfield area. Mary and Mildred Wright bonded immediately. Over an abbreviated period, their relationship evolved into a genuine big and little sister friendship.

Mrs. Wright gave Mary information about the churches (they were Catholic), doctors, hospitals, the Springfield school system, and the positive and negative attitudes among the teachers at the Springfield schools. She gave Mary a rundown on basically the African-American culture in Battle Creek. She told Mary about the beauticians in the area and the available grocery and clothing stores, and where best to shop.

The Moore's were an elderly African-American couple that lived next door to the Wright family. They lived alone in their house, as their children were all adults living on their own. There were two more African-American families that lived in this community; Bishop and Mrs. Harold (Martha McClure Avery-Speights) Speights and the Mayfield family, and they had three girls, Jackie, Audrey, and Tracy, and two girls were the ages of Willis Jr. and Monica.

The Speights' grandson at the time, in 1974, lived in Atlanta, Georgia, when a serial killer had abducted and brutally **murdered** young African-American boys. Bishop and Mrs. Speights' grandson, E. J. Grieg, came to live with them in 1975. My son Kermit and E. J. were the same age, and when they met, they immediately became best friends, and they are still friends today.

When Mary was in a particularly good mood, I would tease her regarding the adjustment she had to make in her shopping habits. She would give me "the look" and then say, "Okay, now, Kalamazoo is only 20 miles away, and don't forget Detroit is really within driving distance. The access Mary had to shop for clothes, shoes, and jewelry items was extremely limited; compared to living in Florissant and the St. Louis areas.

However, collectively the biggest adjustment we, as a family, had to make was being away from our families in St. Louis and East St. Louis.

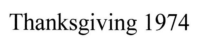

CHAPTER 31

Thanksgiving 1974

I T WAS TWO AND A half months since we moved from Florissant. Now Thanksgiving was on the horizon, one week away. As I observed Mary's demeanor, it appeared that she was feeling a little melancholy. The cause, obviously, to me was that we would spend Thanksgiving apart from our family back home for the first time. The kids also were going to miss our traditional Thanksgiving Day dinner at their grandmamma's house and also going to grandmamma Ruby's house.

I tried to cheer everyone up, assuring them that we would have a wonderful Thanksgiving this year. Mary had begun making plans for preparing a special Thanksgiving dinner. She had her collection of "Family Circle" cookbooks and a new "The Kellogg's cookbook" spread over the dining room table.

A week before Thanksgiving, when I got home from work, Mary was so excited, telling me, "Willis, Mother Drake called and said, "They were coming to visit us for Thanksgiving. Mother Drake, Shirley (Sykes), Queenie (Arcola Drake), Wayne (Gooch), and Crystal (Sykes-Grimmet) were going to drive up Wednesday, Thanksgiving eve and leave Sunday morning going home."

I could see the wheels of Mary's imagination were already spinning. She started giving everybody, including Kermit, tasks to do. This would be Mary's first Thanksgiving to host dinner for our extended family members.

Mary was a fairly good cook in her own right, and she enjoyed cooking. As a "career woman" in nursing, she didn't spend an exorbitant amount of time in the kitchen cooking very often. However, she would prepare a special meal for Thanksgiving and Christmas dinner for our family.

During the ensuing days, suddenly, it was Wednesday, Thanksgiving eve. Birdie and Monica had been alternating looking out the kitchen window all evening, anticipating their cousins' arrival at our house. It was 5:40 pm when my sister Shirley's car pulled into the parking lot of the Fort Custer Apartment Complex. Immediately seeing "Big" Shirley's car, Birdie and Monica ran out to greet them.

Wayne, Queenie, and Crystal filed out of the car, one behind the other. They were laughing, hollering, and hugging as if they had not seen each other in years. It was only two and a half months since we had moved from Florissant.

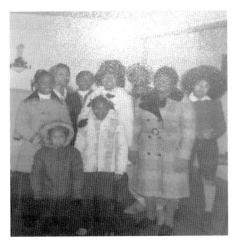

Front row: Kermit Matthew, Crystal; Second row: Monica, (big) Shirley, Mother; Back row: Mary, Willis Jr., Wayne, and Arcola (Queenie)

Now inside the apartment, everybody was extremely emotional, and mother embraced Kermit, Mary, and me. In short order, the ambiance in our apartment was overflowing. Mary displaying her happy smile, asked everybody to make themselves comfortable in our modest abode.

Mother commented, "Mary, the apartment is really nice, and I like how you decorated the walls with beautiful pictures. I always told you that your pictures always seemed to tell a story, and to me, say welcome to our home."

Mary hugged mother again and said, Mother Drake, knowing our apartment passes your approval makes me feel better now. "Sis" (Sister Shirley), come and sit here so we can catch up, girl.

Sitting in the living room, mother, Shirley, Mary, and I were laughing and talking just like in old times. Shirley and Mary were having their side catch-up conversation, as mother and I were talking individually also. The kids were upstairs, and we could hear their voices of joy bouncing off the walls. Kermit was tagging right with Birdie and Wayne.

Mary asked, "are you'll hungry?" Shirley said, girl, nothing has changed; you know I like to eat. They burst out laughing, "yes, I am hungry." Mother said I don't eat that much but I am a little hungry.

Mary called and asked the kids if anyone was hungry. Your dad is going to the Chicken Coop, so let me know what you want to eat. Returning to her chair, "Shirley, the Chicken Coop Snack Shop has the best-fried chicken I have found in the Springfield/Battle Creek area. However, Mother Drake, it can't come close to your fried chicken."

I will call in our order; it should be ready when Willis arrives there. It should only take 20 minutes for him to return home with our food. Birdie and Wayne had on their coats to ride with me. Monica said, "Birdie, you just want to go so you can get the food you want." Laughter resonated loudly in the living room, and Queenie and Chrystal chimed in, saying Birdie, you know that's right.

Shirley was laughing and said it's like they haven't missed a beat from being away from each other. As usual, they still fuss about any and everything, just to be contrary to one another.

Our food was ready when we arrived at the Chicken Coop. I paid for our order, and we were back at the apartment in twenty minutes. Wayne and Birdie carried the food into the house, and Crystal said, "Uncle Willis, the food smells so good. I'm hungry and ready to chow down; how about you, Monica?" Monica, laughing as hard as Crystal was, said, "Crystal, girl, you haven't changed a bit in three months."

You can smell the food and know what's in the bag before seeing it. Queenie, Monica, Birdie, and Wayne were roaring like they always did. Monica suggested that we use paper plates, and Wayne, in his loud voice, said Monica, you just don't want to wash the dishes after we eat. Crystal said, "Monica, you know I will be right there helping you wash the dishes."

The table was set with paper plates, and I blessed the food; as we ate, I observed my nieces and nephew interacting with their cousins, and the apartment felt like back in St. Louis at our mother's house, enjoying our family on a holiday. The kids, including Kermit, were in the dining room, eating and laughing. Mother, Shirley, Mary, and I were in the living room eating and reminiscing about old times.

When we finished eating, Mary clapped her hands and reminded everyone that today was Birdie's 14th birthday. Saying, Mother Drake, I always follow the Drake family tradition, bake the kids a birthday cake. Birdie wanted a yellow cake with chocolate icing and Neapolitan ice cream for his birthday.

Mary brought the cake and ice cream out, Birdie made his "birthday wish," and the family sang happy birthday to him. In the family tradition, he cut the first slice of his birthday cake and scooped up his favorite ice cream. The kids joined in getting their cake and ice cream; and clowning around, and that's how we celebrated Willis Jr.'s fourteenth birthday.

Mary said it was getting late and "I am going to bed. I need plenty of rest so I can get up early in the morning to finish cooking Thanksgiving dinner. Mother said, "Mary, I am going to bed now too."

Shirley and I stayed downstairs talking for hours like we always did when she visited us. Kermit had gone upstairs with Mary, and the older kids were still in the dining room talking when Shirley and I went upstairs to bed.

Thanksgiving Dinner
Traditionally on Thanksgiving Day, mother would invite her children and their families over for Thanksgiving dinner. Mary always prepared a Thanksgiving dinner for our individual family at home, although we went to mother's and also to Mary's parent's home on Thanksgiving Day.

Living in Springfield, Michigan, our family was now in sort-of a "Diaspora" (relocation situation) from our St. Louis family. Now Mary was planning to cook her first Thanksgiving dinner for our extended family. "In her own right, Mary could "burn pretty darn good" in the kitchen herself."

However, she knew there was a different level of expertise compared to what mother could do in the kitchen. Mary was slightly apprehensive about preparing a wonderful Thanksgiving dinner meal.

Mary came downstairs at 8:30 Thanksgiving morning, and she was still energized, and her jubilation was percolating from seeing our family yesterday. She asked if I slept well last night as we kissed, saying she didn't hear me get out of bed this morning.

I rubbed Mary's smiling face and said, "Oh, I got up an hour ago, and you were resting so peacefully, and I didn't want to wake you, so I came downstairs." Walking towards the kitchen, almost laughing, Mary said, "Willis, last night I slept exceptionally well, and I feel totally rested now."

Mary was moving about the kitchen like a confident cook. She was humming and periodically reciting a phrase from a Motown song. She was talking aloud to herself in a musical rhythm, "I will put the turkey in the oven now, the ham in an hour later so that they would be fully cooked by 2:30 pm. Then she shimmied her shoulders and moved to the beat in her humming flow as she slid her feet across the kitchen floor.

Hearing the rhetorical dialogue in the kitchen, I was not sure if Mary was asking me questions and expected a response or not. "Willis, I plan to serve dinner at 2:30 pm, and everyone should be hungry by then; what do you think?"

Then I heard mother coming downstairs. She said good morning and greeted Mary and me with a hug. She exclaimed that she had slept so restfully as if she were home in her own bed. Mary asked, "What do you want for breakfast this morning. Do you still have just your coffee and toast?"

"Mary, I will have one slice of dry toast and a cup of coffee, baby. You know I have to get something in my stomach when I get up in the mornings. Mary, in a minute, I will be in the kitchen to help you prepare your dinner," mother replied.

Mary implored Mother Drake, "you just sit there and enjoy your coffee, relax, and talk to Willis. I have everything under control. I will let you know if I need your help with anything, okay? I plan to serve dinner at 2:30 or 3:00 this afternoon; do you think that is a suitable time to eat?"

Mother took a sip of coffee and said, "yes, Mary, 2:30ish is a perfect time to eat dinner. Are you sure you don't need my help cooking something for dinner? However, I understand too many cooks in the kitchen can be a problem." Mary and I laughed at mother's comment.

Then Mary said, Mother Drake, you would never be a problem being in anybody's kitchen, and certainly not in my kitchen. The laughter increased, and mother sat back and enjoyed her toast and coffee as she and

I talked. I realized that this type of conversation with my mother was a weekly routine when we lived in Florissant.

Standing in the living room, Mary said I could hear the kids stirring around upstairs. As their laughter became more pronounced, mother said, yes, I could hear them too. The girls' voices intensified and got louder, overshadowing the boys' collective voices. Mother said, "I can tell just how happy the kids are to see one another."

"They will be coming downstairs shortly. I hope they don't wake up Shirley. She drove the entire distance from St. Louis yesterday and stayed up late last night talking to you, Willis; I know she was tired, Mary continued. Mother laughed and said, "Mary, when Shirley gets a whiff of the food you are cooking; I know she will wake up and will be ready to eat."

It was 11:15 am when the three girls came downstairs. As usual, when Monica and Crystal were together, it was like a perpetual comedy show. The two of them laughed all the time. Monica came straight to her grandmother with a big smile and gave her a lingering hug. Saying good morning, grandmamma, did you sleep well last night? I hope our giggling and girl talk didn't keep you awake.

Still hugging Monica, mother said, "I miss seeing your pretty smile "Miss Renee" (That's the nickname her grandmother called Monica). No, I didn't hear anything last night, and I slept like a baby."

Monica said, "grandmamma, I have to go help momma, and my responsibility is to set the dinner table with the appropriate tableware (plates, glasses, napkins, and silverware). Momma wants everything perfect for Thanksgiving dinner. Momma constantly reminds me that I am to always use proper table etiquette.

With her magnetic smile, Monica said, "Grandmamma, I can't use paper plates for dinner like I did last night. Grandmamma smiled and said, "Your mother is teaching you right," and "you should get Crystal to help you. She needs to practice how to set a formal dinner table too."

Crystal and Arcola (Queenie) hugged their grandmother, asking how she felt, and engaged in small talk and chitchatted with her. They acknowledged me with a hug, and Queenie said, "Uncle Willis, I didn't intend to sleep so late. Immediately, her attention switched as she said to Crystal, "you are right, everything smells really good, girl, and it's making me hungry."

Queenie, with her facetious laugh, said, "Uncle Willis, don't think I came to visit you and Aunt Mary just to sleep and eat." Queenie then rushed to the kitchen, said hi to Aunt Mary, and hugged her.

Right on cue, Wayne, Birdie, and Kermit Matthew came downstairs and into the living room. Shirley came downstairs in her housecoat. She said good morning to everybody and sat on the couch. Kermit, hanging with the big boys, was hesitant to give his mother a big hug as he normally did. However, he rushed to hug his grandmother and Aunt Shirley. When we lived in Florissant, Shirley would keep Kermit so he could play with her German Shepherd dog, Smoke.

With everyone now downstairs, the house was filled with chatter and laughter. Sitting on the couch, I was observing my mother, sister, nieces, nephew, and children sharing their love, and I was subconsciously reveling in how blessed our family was on this Thanksgiving Day.

An eight-hour drive from St. Louis was not a deterrent to keep our families from getting together for a traditional Thanksgiving Day dinner. Living away from St. Louis for the first time and now having our family together here in Springfield, Michigan, to celebrate our first Thanksgiving dinner here was a true blessing.

As the dinner hour drew closer, Monica was helping her mother with a few incidental preparations for dinner. After the turkey and ham had cooled, I carved the turkey and sliced the ham. Monica put the serving platters on the dinner table as the ten of us prepared to eat a blessed Thanksgiving Day dinner.

Mary had prepared a scrumptious meal that included turkey and ham, cornbread dressing, giblets gravy, macaroni and cheese, green beans, potato salad, and cranberry sauce, and Mary made yeast rolls. We would have the cake and ice cream left from Birdie's 14th birthday for dessert.

We all sat at the dining room table, and each of us at the dinner table individually said a Bible verse or what we were thankful for. I gave special thanks for allowing our families to come together for this blessed Thanksgiving Day. We then dug in to eat, and there was less talking going on now.

The warmth and happiness were shared amongst us, and as I observed the cousins, they acted more like sisters and brothers. They were eating dinner and teasing and joking with one another, which reflected their close relationship. Most of all, their visit eradicated the notion that our family was far away from "home."

After dinner that night at 7:30, the kids went to the skating rink. Wayne asked his mother if he could drive to the skating rink. That it was only 10 minutes from the apartment. Shirley looked at Mary for a silent concurrence, which Mary acknowledged, and Shirley said okay, Wayne, you can drive; drive carefully, and don't be speeding. Also, don't try to show off at the skating rink. I know you and what you are thinking.

Mary, laughing, asked what time is skating over. Birdie said, at 11:30, mom, it will only take us ten or fifteen minutes to drive home.

Mary said Shirley, do you remember when we went skating at the East St. Louis skating rink? I could really roller skate, and you could skate much better than I did. Our kids don't know what roller-shaking is all about. Mary stood up, saying, I could skate backward almost as well as I could skate forward. Shirley said roller skating was fun when we were growing up. Monica was laughing as the kids left the apartment.

Mother said, "no matter how old I get, that same message is echoed when your kids go out at nighttime. Mary laughed and said, "Mother

Drake, that day is approaching for us now that Birdie just turned 14 years old. Monica will be right behind him in a couple of years too.

Kermit was content being nestled next to his grandmother, who was hugging him, and his aunt Shirley on his other side. The four adults talked about everything that was going on in St. Louis and Florissant areas. Shirley told us how Chad Hanna, Wayne's friend, an African-American family living in the subdivision where she lived. Wayne had established a great friendship with Chad, his brother Alex, his sister, and the Hanna family during their school years. Chad and Wayne remained lifelong friends.

We were still laughing and talking, and Kermit was sleeping on the couch. We heard the front door open, and the kids were back from the skating rink. They obviously had a super time, and now we had to listen to Wayne's account of how he "skated rings around those dudes, and he was giving free lessons with his spellbinding skating demonstrations."

We were laughing and enjoying listening to Wayne's alleged skating prowess. However, Queenie, Crystal, and Monica debated his account's accuracy. Birdie naturally sided with Wayne. There was a back and forth of what was the truth between the cousins' recollections. In short order, we all headed to bed.

Friday and Saturday
There were few tourist attractions in the Battle Creek area. However, "Friday afternoon, we visited the "Turkey Farm," which mother enjoyed, but the kids were totally bored at the turkey farm.

On Saturday, everybody was chilling-out. The kids were doing their thing, just hanging out upstairs. The gaiety among them was prevalent throughout the house. As the evening approached, the kids started to wind down. It was as if they knew there would be an emotional letdown Sunday morning when they had to leave to go back home.

Mother, Shirley, Mary, and I sat in the liver room talking, mostly about how Mary liked living in Springfield; and how she was adjusting to the

Battle Creek area overall. Mary said, "she was still house hunting. However, we wanted to find a house in Springfield, so the kids could remain in the Springfield school district.

Also, she might consider returning to work after the first of the year. Shirley said, "Mary, after working for so many years, I don't think I could stay home all day being a homemaker." Working is part of my daily routine now. "Shirley, I have the apartment decorated and organized the way I want it now. Maybe I will plan to start working again after the new year as soon as January or February."

The conversation regarding Mary considering working was the first firm indication that I had heard her say she was interested in getting a job after the New Year. Now it was evening, about 4:30 pm, and Mary called upstairs for the kids to come so we could eat dinner. We had Thanksgiving leftovers, which tasted as good now as they did on Thanksgiving.

After dinner, Mary packed slices of turkey and ham for the family to take on the trip back to St. Louis. They could make sandwiches, and they had water and soft drinks to take with them, so they would not have to stop for food going home.

That night in bed, Mary said, "In almost a whisper. "Willis, I feel like one of Mother Drake's daughters, not like a daughter-in-law. You know we have an incredibly special family." My eyes were looking up at the ceiling; "baby, I feel like a son to your mom and dad; and a big brother to your brothers and sisters. We have truly been blessed as a family. Holding Mary in my arms, we finally dozed off to sleep.

I woke up before 6:00 o'clock Sunday morning, knowing our family would be returning home to St. Louis in an hour. Like a flash of lightning, now everyone was up and scurrying around getting dressed. It was now 7:00 am, and mother, Shirley, and the kids were saying their goodbyes with short hugs and happy tears in their eyes.

They left the apartment to get on the road and head home. I said a silent prayer for their safe travels on the highway. Our apartment that entire day was a solemn place as we floated back to reality, having experienced the wonderful Thanksgiving weekend with our family. However, I knew the memories of the joy we had this Thanksgiving would swing our emotions to a positive place going forward.

NOTE

Following the first year living in Springfield, we got settled there. As a routine, we would travel home most years during the kids' school Christmas breaks. The family would get together at my parent's home for Christmas dinner. The Christmas dinner meal that mother prepared was her gift to her children and their families. She prepared everything herself and resisted help from anyone to cook the food.

Interestingly enough, in 1983, I asked Mary how she felt if she and I would prepare Christmas dinner this year. Therefore, mother would not have all that demanding work cooking the meal. Mary immediately replied, "Willis, do you think Mother Drake would turn over her kitchen to me, so I could cook Christmas dinner?"

Initially, I laughed because I didn't make the correlation between mother not having to work so hard preparing a large dinner meal; with her relinquishing control of "her kitchen" to someone else.

I now understood the gravity of mother turning over her kitchen to Mary. When I asked mother if it was okay for Mary to prepare the Christmas dinner this year, without hesitation, she said, "yes, that will be fine."

The climax of that Christmas was when we video recorded mother's and Mary's conversation, discussing mother turning over her kitchen to Mary. I recall the poignant words spoken between the two of them!

Mary—"Mother Drake, when Willis told me you agreed to turn over your kitchen to me, to cook Christmas dinner, I asked Willis are you sure mother Drake said yes?"

Mother—laughing and said, "Mary, when Willis asked me if you could prepare Christmas dinner, I had to really think a minute, but

I quickly said yes. Mary, you are the first person I ever turned my kitchen over to."

Mary—was laughing now also, and she said, "Mother Drake, I know it's not easy to turn your kitchen over to anyone. When Willis said it was okay for me to cook Christmas dinner, and you had turned your kitchen over to me, I knew I truly was like one of your daughters."

Mother—said with a serious soft tone in her voice, "You are my daughter."

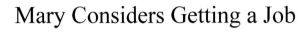

CHAPTER 32

Mary Considers Getting a Job

Aᴼ FTER THANKSGIVING, FOR SOME REASON, Mary's focus seemed to shift towards going back to work. I don't know if there were conversations during Thanksgiving that ignited her interest or if it was remembering her effort to complete nursing school that motivated her.

For six years before Kermit was born, Mary was a working mother pursuing her professional nursing career. With our family structure of working parents with two children, Mary had morphed into excellently performing her incredibly challenging dual responsibilities as a mother, wife, and professional career woman.

When Kermit was born, Mary became a full-time stay-at-home mom until Kermit was two and a half years old. Mary's innate yearnings to resume her nursing career heightened at that time, and she decided to work part-time on weekends. This was basically appeasement, and it provided the gratification that Mary needed. She worked weekends for a year and a half prior to us moving to Springfield, Michigan.

During her engaging conversations with Shirley and mother during their Thanksgiving visit, Mary's desire to return to work became evident. One evening we were in the family room watching TV, and fortuitously the conversation of Mary working again came up. She said, "Hey babe, I'm thinking of returning to work after the New Year begins."

She stated, which she correctly assessed, "that Birdie and Monica had adjusted well in the Springfield community, and Kermit was also settled into his kindergarten schedule. If I work the evening shift at a hospital, I can still take Kermit to school in the mornings. However, we will have to put Kermit in daycare for a few hours in the evenings until you get off work."

Looking at her, I could tell Mary's intent was to work again. I reminded Mary that we were in solid shape financially and she did not need to start working again to earn money. Mary said, "Willis, my motivation to work is for my professional and personal desires, and there are no ancillary reasons. I know you will always take care of our family."

We agreed that Mary would plan to start working soon. So during dinner, she discussed with the kids her plan to get a job and start working at a hospital shortly. Therefore, everybody will have to pitch in and do their part in helping around the house. The laughter around the dinner table grew louder as we finished our dinner.

During the ensuing days, Mary discussed with her friend Mildred (Wright) her interest in getting a job. Mildred suggested that Mary should inquire at "The United States Department of Veterans Affairs (VA) hospital." It was located at 5500 Armstrong Road, Battle Creek, MI., only ten minutes from where you live. Mary chose the VA hospital as her primary interest in applying for a job.

Daycare for Kermit

Mary was confident she would get a job as a registered nurse when she submitted her application. However, she first needed to find the best daycare center for Kermit to attend a few hours after school. With Mildred Wright's help, Mary found a daycare center on Washington Avenue, five minutes from the Federal Center where I worked.

Before Mary had a job, Mary and I visited the certified daycare center, and placed our name on the waiting list for a future space for Kermit.

The owner and daycare instructors were very professional, and the day-care facility was clean and very well organized.

1975 Mary Hired at the VA Battle Creek Medical Center:
With her enthusiasm to get a job, Mary applied for a Registered Nurse's (RN) position at the VA Hospital the next week. The following week she had an in-person interview for the RN position.

The morning of her interview, when I was leaving for work, "I wished Mary good luck on your interview today, babe. I am sure you will "ace" the interview."

When I got home from work, Mary was upbeat as she recounted how her job interview had gone. She smiled as she told me that she felt very positive when she completed her interview. That there were three head nurses participating in the interview, and I answered all of their questions with detailed substance. I would just wait and see what the results are.

In less than two weeks, the VA personnel office verified Mary's nurse's credentials and qualifications. The VA personnel office notified Mary that she was hired as a Registered Nurse at the Battle Creek VA Medical Center, and she started working in early February 1975.

Mary cautiously integrated into the VA nursing staff, getting oriented with the VA hospital culture as an African-American registered nurse. She was one of only a few African-American registered nurses working at the Battle Creek VA Medical Center.

Mary was a dedicated and professional nurse. Most of the issues, or concerns, centered around any unwarranted mis-behavior to the VA pa-tients. Mary's position was to treat all patients respectfully and provide them with the best care. She made her position clear and known to the nursing attendants. In short order, Mary became known as a voice for the patients.

Mary working the evening shift provided us with some conveniences, but there were also inconveniences. I would stay awake every night until

Mary got home. Regardless of how tired I was, I stayed awake until she was safely in the house. Overall, we balanced our work schedules and personal time very well, and we treasured our time together.

CHAPTER 33

⬦

Buying a House

⬦

MARY "MULTITASKED" IN HER ROLES as a wife, working mother, and managing the household with teenagers and a five year older. However, her focus on finding the right house for our family to buy did not waver.

Cecil and Gerri Black gave Mary's contact information to Virginia, their real estate agent. Mary and I decided the kids would remain in the Springfield School District. Therefore, we would buy a house in the city of Springfield. Mary always enjoyed looking at houses; she looked at houses in Springfield and the surrounding communities independent of a realtor. There was one house we considered buying but it did not work out.

However, when I was spiritually guided, it seemed that we always came out on top, notwithstanding the situation. I had prayed that we would find the right house for our family in the Springfield community.

A few weeks later, Mary called me at work in the early afternoon, and she sounded excited. "Willis, Virginia, just called about a house for sale located in Springfield that was just listed with their agency. Virginia will not list the property (house) for sale until she shows us the house first.

We can see the house this evening, and Virginia will meet us there at 5:00 o'clock. The house is located at 31 Royal Road, Springfield, MI. It is in that exclusive area of Springfield where Mildred and Jim Wright live. The house is also around the corner from where Bishop and Mrs. Harold Speights live."

When I got home, Mary and the kids were ready to go see the house. I cautioned them to slow down, it only takes 10 minutes to drive there, and we have plenty of time. Also, Mary, if you really like the house, just "be cool." Don't overreact with excitement in front of Virginia that you want to buy the house.

Mary gave me that evil eye look like I was schooling her as if she was an inexperienced real estate consumer. We got in the car, and 12 minutes later, we arrived at the house. It was a half block from the Valley View Springfield Elementary School, where Kermit attended school, and a block and a half from the Springfield Junior High School, where Monica went to school.

Virginia was in her car, parked in the driveway. I parked next to her vehicle, and, standing in the driveway, we greeted one another. Mary introduced Virginia to our children, and we all entered the house. When Mary and I first stepped across the threshold, we immediately looked at one another, not saying a word. Somehow, simultaneously, we knew this house was to be our home.

We didn't have to painstakingly look throughout the house with great intensity. The kids were excited, checking out every room in the house. They started picking out which bedroom was going to be theirs. The backyard, the fireplace, etc., was very nice. This was the second time in buying a house, that it had been demonstrated that we just need to be patient and know everything will be all right!

Observing the smile on Mary's face let me know that she was satisfied with this house. There were physical similarities between this house and the house we owned in Florissant. The carpet in the living room and dining room in this house was the exact type of carpet we had in our home in Florissant.

The house had a brick front with aluminum siding on the sides and back of the house. Inside, it had three bedrooms upstairs, a living room and a formal dining room, and a large family room with a double glass sliding door that exited to the patio in the backyard. The backyard was large, and there was a sizable front yard as well.

It had a large, fully finished basement with a laundry room, a fourth bedroom, a workshop, and a gas sauna room for taking a steam (sauna) bath, and there was sufficient storage space. There was an attached one-car garage and one and a half bathrooms. This house, the same as our home in Florissant, I believe was made available to us resulting from fortuity, if not by fate.

It was obvious that Mary, the kids, and I really liked this house. Mary and I made an offer on the house that evening. Virginia, the realtor, said she would notify the homeowners of our offer and let us know if they would accept it.

The next evening when Monica came home from school, "Dad, my classmate Leslie Heichler, told me her father said that the "Drake family was buying our house." Monica, if the homeowners (Heichler's) accepted our offer, we would be moving into that house soon. The following day Virginia informed us that our offer had been accepted and we should expect to close within 30 days.

Moved from Fort Custer Apartment:
We purchased our home eight months after moving to Springfield, Michigan. When we had access to the house, our family went to the house, and we formed a circle holding hands, with the Bible in the center, and I read the 23rd Psalm. Those instructions had been my mother's original guidance to me in blessing the first house we purchased in Florissant.

Now the kids were older, and Willis Jr. and Monica packed their bedrooms to move into our house. During that week, we all helped clean the house, and I rented a U-Haul truck and moved into our new house on Saturday.

Again we had help from Our reliable friends, Cecil, and Gerri Black, and help from a few of Willis Jr.'s young high school friends. We moved from the apartment and into our new house without any problems. At the end of the day, all the furniture was in the rooms where it belonged. I returned the U-Haul rental truck, and I returned to our own home.

I entered the house, and Mary greeted me at the door; I saw the happiness on her face now that we owned our home. She said, "Willis, I am able to use all the furniture we own; and not have to store it in the basement. We settled into our new home very comfortably. Our house was located in the "upscale community in the Springfield area."

However, there were a few families in this community that had a sadity or snooty attitude. There was an "air about them," giving the impression or thinking they were better than someone else. We interacted with the families in this community more so, whereas we had not done so with the families in the Fort Custer apartment complex.

Within a week, Mary, the kids, and I had the house in shape resembling the standards of our home when we lived in Florissant. Everybody was happy, and now Mary was pleased to put the work effort into her own home instead of a rented apartment.

Everything continued falling in place as if it was intended. Mary was still working the evening 3:30 pm to 11:30 pm shift at the VA Medical Center. Moving to our home at 31 Royal Road only added five minutes to her commute to work.

Our home was closer to the Valley View Elementary School, 960 Avenue A, where Kermit went to kindergarten. The school was only five minutes for him to walk to and from school. Mary would drop him off and meet him in the school's playground area after school, and they walked home together.

Kermit's Daycare
We enrolled Kermit in the daycare center located on Washington Avenue, near the Federal Center where I worked. Kermit had been attending the daycare center for two weeks, and it had worked out very well. Mary would take him to the daycare on her way to work, and I would pick him up when I got off work.

The third week when I picked Kermit up from the daycare, he had been crying. I asked him what was wrong, and the daycare instructor intervened and said, Mr. Drake, Kermit would not take his nap as he was supposed to, and he got upset.

Riding home, Kermit said, "dad, I laid down on my palette like the other kids, but I didn't go to sleep. The teacher was upset when I couldn't sleep, and she spanked me, which is why I was crying."

When Mary got home from work that night, I told her what had happened at the daycare, and she was livid. It was truly fortunate that Mary had not picked Kermit up from the daycare. Otherwise, she would have returned to the daycare and taken that teacher to task.

The next day Mary told Mildred Wright about the incident yesterday at the daycare. Mrs. Wright told Mary to bring Kermit down to her house when she went to work, and he could stay with her, and I could pick him up when I got home from work.

How perfect could it be that Mrs. Wright was right on time when we needed her? She would not accept any payment as compensation for the two hours Kermit stayed at her house. She told Mary how excited she was to have Kermit around. They would read and work on his numbers (math) counting, and she said he is really smart. She enjoyed having Kermit around her.

When Kermit was eight or nine years old, Mrs. Wright's brother, Dennis Louis Joyner (Kermit called him Uncle Dennis), arranged for Kermit and me to attend a Notre Dame football game in South Bend, IN. Mrs. Wright's younger brother, Lemuel Martin Joyner, was on the Notre Dame teaching staff, and he got excellent tickets for Kermit and me to attend the football game.

Until the fourth grade, Kermit continued going to Mrs. Wright's home after school. She allowed two neighborhood kids, who were Kermit's closest friends, E J Grieg, and John Allen, to play outside with Kermit. When Kermit turned ten years old, he was responsible enough that he no longer went to Mrs. Wright's house after school.

When Kermit was attending Springfield Middle and Junior High School, he periodically would stop by Mrs. Wright's house to see her. Kermit and Mrs. Wright had a special bond that played a prominent role in Kermit's growth during elementary school.

Mary's Family Reunion

When we purchased our house in June of 1975, Mary agreed to host her Family Reunion in Springfield, Michigan. It was a small gathering of family members that attended the reunion. However family came from East St. Louis, Illinois, St. Louis, Missouri, Detroit, Michigan, and Marion, Indiana.

The reunion served as a building block to connect the three generations from Mary's mother's generation to Mary's generation and the next generation represented by our children's generation.

Ruby Smith-Byas, Mildred Smith-Thomas (Mary's Aunt Biddy), Lovie Austin Banks, Ethel Ard, and Addie Estelle White were of the older generation; Mary Ann Byas-Drake, Paul Tolden, and Linda Turner represented the current generation; Willis Drake Jr., Monica Renee Drake, and Kermit Matthew Drake represented the next generation, who were the younger family members.

For the reunion, Mrs. Ruby Smith-Byas, Paul Tolden and his wife Irene Tolden, and Linda Turner traveled from East St. Louis, IL.; Mildred Thomas (Aunt Biddy) traveled from St. Louis, MO; Mary's cousins

Lovie Austin Banks; and Ethel Ard traveled from Detroit, MI; Addie Estelle White traveled from Marion, Indiana; and our family lives in Springfield, MI.

The generational family matriarchs were obviously pleased going forward with the family legacy being in the hands of the next generation's younger family members; that would elevate the family going forward. Moreover, Mary was humbled as her family offered accolades of her and our family. It was an opportunity for the extended family to also "christen" our home as they expressed their approval of us having a "beautiful" home. Mary was pleased that her family was satisfied with her station in life.

Mary, the host city's hostess, arranged activities for the family members to participate in during the weekend. Our home was the place for the out-of-town guests to gather, socialize, and interact with the family for our planned activities and to feel like they were at home.

Mary's mother, Aunt Biddy, and their first cousins, Love, Ethel, and Estelle, had not seen one another in several years. I was fascinated just sitting, listening, and observing the ladies reminisce about their childhood, and hearing the stories they told were fascinating, enjoyable, and entertaining.

We went to dinner at a favorite local restaurant Saturday evening. After dinner, we returned to our home and just kicked back, and Mary's cousin Estelle was very comical. She told stories about their young childhood that was hilarious. The family gathering was "out of sight" as the family share time together, and Mary was pleased that her family had asked us to host the reunion.

Mary was pleased that her mother and Aunt Biddy, and our family members complimented her on how she had decorated our house. Everyone was able to relax and socialize comfortably in our home. At the same time, Mary's cousin, Paul, and her were reminiscing about their childhood. It was a festive atmosphere, and Paul added his unique humor.

All family members that were traveling returned home safely. After the reunion for weeks, Mary talked about how she enjoyed seeing all her family members, especially her cousins she grew up with.

CHAPTER 34

───── ◇ ─────

Mary's Bachelor (BSN) and Master of Science (MSN) Degrees in Nursing

───── ◇ ─────

W HEN WE LIVED IN FLORISSANT, Missouri, Mary had seriously contemplated pursuing her BSN **(Bachelor of Science in Nursing)** degree. It was during this time, however, that she wanted to have another baby. She was slightly conflicted, as she desired to get her college degree; however, her yearning to have another child superseded her aspirations for getting her college degree at this time.

As Kermit advanced to being a toddler, Mary's ambition and thirst to earn her college degree never waned. That constant flicker of light to get her college degree remained strong in her spirit and consciousness.

When we moved to Springfield, Michigan, Kermit was almost five years old. Willis Jr. and Monica were teenagers and had become more self-sufficient and reliable. As a result, Mary's desire to get her BSN degree was buoyed significantly. Mary getting her nursing degree, remained prominent in our discussions in our normal routine conversations.

I am not sure if Mary's quest to obtain her **college** degree qualifies as an "Episode" in her life; or a situation that was destined to happen.

Figuratively speaking, she maintained a fire within her that was inextinguishable that she had to satisfy.

This particular night, I heard the outside garage door open and retracting up. Then I heard the inside garage door open coming into the house, and I knew Mary was home safely. For some reason, tonight was slightly different.

Mary was always quiet when she came into the house, so she didn't wake up the kids. Tonight there appeared to be no emphasis on her being quiet. She was walking rapidly from the family room, down the hallway, and to our bedroom. There seemed to be a sense of urgency about her. I could hear the squishing sound of her feet moving up and down in her cushioned nurse's shoes.

In a matter of seconds, she was standing at my bedside whispering, "Willis, baby, are you awake?" Raising my head from my pillow, I laughed softly and replied humorously, "baby, don't be silly. You know I am awake and talking with you now." She kissed me as she always did.

She said, "Man," you know what I mean. Baby, I hope you are not very sleepy; I want to talk, okay? I sat up in bed, and it was obvious that Mary had something serious she wanted to talk about. Trying to be attentive, I said, "come here, girl, tell me what's on your mind, as I slid over and made room for her to sit on the bed.

"Willis, over the past few years, we discussed me getting my BSN degree, and unfortunately, I procrastinated for one reason or another. However, I decided to start working this year to get my nursing degree.

Mary stood up, stressed her arms in the air, and started getting ready for bed." It was obvious that she was still in a talkative frame of mind. As she was getting undressed, she said, "baby, I started my VA job in 1975. Within a few years, I realized that the standard three-year diploma nurse would be overcome career-wise by nurses with a four-year BSN college degree.

She was talking aloud softly, in a thinking mode, as she continued getting ready for bed. She was not necessarily talking to me, but possibly hearing her "verbal articulation" was for her own assurance and validation. Possibly she needed to convince herself that she was ready to embark on this tremendous undertaking to earn her college degree.

Now with her pajamas on, Mary slid under the covers as she got in bed. She was still talking as I imagined what thoughts were floating around her mind. She said baby; I have determined the college courses required for me to earn a BSN degree. Also, I have identified the courses I can take at a local college. Mary sighed as she was now resting comfortably in bed, and finally, she was all talked out, and we went to sleep.

Our normal daily routine continued as time passed quickly, fleeting week after week. Kermit was in the fourth grade, and Mary was working the day shift. She had all her ducks in a row as she prepared to start classes at the local Kellogg Community College (KCC), located at 450 North Avenue, Battle Creek, MI, for the January 1978 semester. KCC was only fifteen minutes from our house.

However, when she exhausted the courses available at KCC, she enrolled at Western Michigan University (WMU) to take classes. She now had to travel twenty miles to Kalamazoo, MI, 30 minutes from our house in Springfield.

Mary had class two nights a week. Joking, I would say, "Mary as mother used to tell me, don't bring a grade in this house below a "C." Mary would laugh and give me that look, "indicating for me to shut my mouth and be quiet."

As the semester was ending, Mary was upbeat and confident that she had earned at least a "B" grade in her classes. She also had been preparing for the past several months to take the credit by examination tests for college credit. Baby, I have paid my test fee, which is non-refundable. I am scheduled to take four college examination tests in the next two weeks at WMU.

Willis, I will be studying this week, brushing up, in preparation for two tests this coming Saturday and another two the following Saturday. My test results will determine if I receive in-class course credit, via the "credit by examination" process. This process will accelerate my earning a BSN degree sooner.

Saturday morning, Mary left the house to take her tests, looking extremely confident, and I also felt that she would do well on her tests.

When Mary returned home that evening, she described the tests as incredibly challenging, but she was confident she had done well. As the week rolled around, she got ready to take the last two tests on the upcoming Saturday. Returning home, similar to her initial reaction last Saturday, she was confident that she had also done well on these tests.

We all were waiting for Mary's test results to come. At dinner one evening, Mary said, "I checked, and the closest university to where we live that offered a four-year BSN nursing degree is the University of Michigan (U of M) at Ann Arbor, Michigan.

So I contacted the U of M admittance office, and I confirmed that their school of nursing would accept my "nurses' work experience for college credit; and my "credit by examination" test results, as well." I received my grades from Western Michigan University, notifying me that I passed all four tests with an A or B grade.

Now I will forward my documentation package to the U of M for evaluation. It will include my educational documentation, dating back to Lincoln high school in 1958. My Southern Illinois University (SIU), Kellogg's community college, and Western Michigan University college credits, plus my ten years of work experience as a registered nurse."

Two weeks later, the U of M sent Mary a letter notifying her that they had ascribed college credit for her work experience and her "credit by examination" results towards a BSN degree in their nursing school program. Her tenacity had culminated in meeting all benchmark requirements to obtain college credit toward a U of M BSN degree.

Mary said that "the dynamics have changed considerably at the VA hospital over the past few years. The young nurses coming into the VA workforce now have their BSN degrees. Therefore, in the future, the degreed RNs would likely be promoted first within the VA system.

Now more than anything, I want a college degree for my personal achievement and better job security at the VA hospital." That night, she declared she would get her BSN degree and was laser-focused. There was no doubt in my mind that Mary would be successful in this endeavor, earning her BSN degree.

The weekend came very quickly, and at the breakfast table, Mary said, I told you all a few days ago that I have been accepted at the U of M to get my college degree. Before I start my classes, I want to let you'll know how truly blessed I am.

Mary's words seemed to elevate everyone's response to a joyous mood. Now we were finishing breakfast celebrating "momma" (Mary), who was destined and determined. She stated, as a matter of fact, "I will begin classes in January to start the winter semester at the U of M in Ann Arbor."

This Saturday morning was different from most. Monica volunteered to clean up the kitchen when we had finished eating breakfast. She said, "okay, Birdie and Kermit, you can leave the kitchen, so I can clean up." Mary and I exited the kitchen, retreating to our normal Saturday activities. However, we retreated to the living room, which we very seldom used, so we could have a private conversation regarding her starting college.

Pursuing BSN College Degree
Mary's feet were planet on a solid foundation in her quest to earn her degree. In the midst of her quest to earn her college degree, every other aspect of our daily lives continued. In June 1979, Willis Jr. graduated from Springfield High School. He then attended the local Kellogg Community College.

Monica was a junior at Springfield High School, and Kermit Matthew attended Springfield Elementary School. As a family, we had our routine worked out, as Mary's work schedule was convenient and accommodating for her. She was able to participate in every meaningful milestone and activity the kids were involved with.

Mary was balancing her activities to start college that year, and she was helping Monica navigate through her senior year of high school and prepare for college. In 1981, Mary enrolled at the University of Michigan (U of M), taking classes on campus in Ann Arbor, Michigan. She had to focus on driving 136 miles round-trip to Ann Arbor three days a week. Her long commute was just a slight imposition to earn her U of M BSN degree.

Mary had to travel highway I-94 for that long distance and often returned home late at night. For Mary's safety and my peace of mind, we went to the Chevrolet (Chevy) Dealership to purchase her a small compact car. That type of vehicle would be easier for her to drive and handle.

Mary saw this very sharp-looking coco brown, four-door Chevy sedan. Smiling from ear to ear, she said baby, this is the car I want. Her statement was very definitive, and I also agree with her selection of that automobile. We purchased the new car she could drive with dependability and confidence, traveling to and from the U of M.

I teased Mary that she had better be careful, driving her "fly car" on the U of M campus. We both laughed as we arrived home and pulled into the garage.

Walking into the house, Monica and Kermit Matthew blurted out, "momma, what kind of car did you get?" With a big smile on her face, she said, "please, first, let me get my coat off and sit down." She intentionally took longer than necessary to hang up her coat as she teased the kids with her silence.

Mary proceeded to describe her Coco-colored Nova Chevy automobile down to the finest detail. She said I would pick up my car in two days. She put her arm around Monica's shoulder, who was sitting next to her mother on the couch. Without skipping a beat, she said, "Monica, don't get any idea that you will be driving my car." Laughing, she continued describing the car in detail.

As the evening faded into night, Mary and I continued talking. She was excited about taking classes at the Ann Arbor campus. She recognized that this undertaking was a significant challenge. Her classmates basically were resident students living on campus, and they did not have to commute to get to their classes. Mary approached her commuting situation with the same determination she had in the past years in pursuing her BSN degree.

Mary's school year started, and she had an enjoyable and successful first year as a student on the campus of the U of M. Now, as her semester was ending, in June 1981, Monica graduated from Springfield High School. She had been accepted at Western Michigan University (WMU). As parents, Mary and I had orchestrated and arranged for Monica to enter WMU in September for the school's fall semester.

At this point, Mary wanted to concentrate and focus on getting Monica situated firmly to begin her first year of college. Monica going off to college occurred as we had anticipated. It seemed that the summer had evaporated, and almost immediately, Mary and I had loaded up our two vehicles with Monica's belongings. We were then off to drop our daughter at Western Michigan University, twenty miles away in Kalamazoo, Michigan.

For whatever reason, Monica struggled during her first year at WMU and was on academic probation. She had to take a summer class to bolster her Grade Point Average (GPA) to return to WMU for her sophomore year.

Mary was determined to help get Monica straighten out academically in college. During the summer of 1982, Mary suggested to Monica that they take a summer class together, and they enrolled in an "elective class" at WMU. Mary wanted to demonstrate firsthand to Monica how to apply herself to be successful in college. When they completed the class, Monica said she got a "B" grade for the class; but "momma" got an "A" in the class."

Passing that summer class with a "B" grade, Monica was eligible to start her sophomore year at WMU" without probation." Mary also earned additional course credit for her college transcript. Mary's dedication to that summer was primarily to inspire her daughter Monica to know what it would take "for her" to get a college education. Mary's outlook and expectations for Monica's college prospects for the next semester were high.

Overall, Mary's pursuit of obtaining her BSN degree was not a smooth, uneventful journey. One evening returning home from school, she had a serious accident driving from Ann Arbor. It was late October or early November, and it was freezing outside in the late evening. It was dark out, and it was also the **"Deer rutting season." As a result, the Deer were roaming everywhere, including across the highway."**

I was home watching television, and the phone rang a little past 6:30 pm. I answered the phone "hello." Immediately, I heard Mary's voice say, "Willis, I had an accident tonight on the highway driving home. Baby, I am fine!"

Immediately my voice elevated, asking, "Mary, baby, are you okay? I repeated myself, and the redundancy of my question rang out in my mind. Mary was composed as she responded, "Willis, physically, I am doing fine now. I was not injured, and there is not a scratch on me. However, baby, for an instant, I was scared and thought I might die. Then she started crying.

Willis, "When the car started skidding off down into the medium of the highway, I just prayed. I gripped the steering wheel tighter and would not let go; I closed my eyes and prayed. Willis, I knew the car was going to turn over. Then it came to a sudden stop in the medium of the highway. I opened my eyes, and I felt like a miracle had just happened. My prayers were answered. Baby, emotionally, I am shaken up a little, but otherwise, I am fine."

My emotions had intensified, and I could tell from the sound of Mary's voice that she had been crying heavily. There was a pause, and Mary gave a big sigh (I could hear as she exhaled her breath), and she started to explain what the police officer had surmised. "The officer said, "He thought that a car hit a Deer crossing the highway, and oil from the car, spilled onto the highway.

That caused a frozen oil slick on the highway, making the highway surface very slick." "Willis, I was not driving fast. However, the highway at that particular spot was like a sheet of ice. My car skidded and spun into the medium of the highway so quickly."

She paused, and again, I asked, "baby are you okay." At that point, she became emotional and started crying again. Through her sobbing, she managed to tell me the car is not drivable; it was almost bent in half. Regaining her composure, she stated that the first police officer who arrived on the scene of the accident; said, "lady, if your car had rolled over, you probably would have been seriously injured or killed. You are so fortunate that you were not injured."

At this point, my emotions also surfaced. "I thank God that He watches over you as you travel the highways." Mary said, "Willis, looking at my car, it is unbelievable that I don't have a scratch on me."

Willis, the tow truck just arrived. Will you tell the driver where to tow the car? I informed the driver that we are AAA service members and that he should tow the car to the Chevy car dealership; located on Dickerson at Capital Avenues in Battle Creek. Mary was able to ride with the tow truck driver to the dealership location.

I was waiting at the Chevy Dealership lot when the tow truck arrived. I helped Mary from the tow truck, and it was obvious that she was still shaken up by the accident. I embraced her in my arms and kissed her, letting her know I was so thankful she was not injured.

I looked at the crooked and bent metal on the car. I repeatedly whispered in Mary's ear, "I am so thankful you are safe." However, in reality, we both were spiritually uplifted. Looking at the car wreckage, we both understood that for Mary not to have a scratch on her, it had to be a "Spiritual" presence in the midst of that accident that protected her.

Driving home, Mary had her head resting on my shoulder. This was a habit she had from when we were first dating. Reflectively, Mary said, "Willis, just thinking about you and the kids, I truly know how blessed I am." Arriving home, we sat in the car for a few minutes so Mary could collect herself emotionally before going into the house and seeing the kids.

We entered the house, and Monica and Kermit converged at the door and met their mother; both hugged her, claiming some part of her body to embrace. Birdie was more composed, and he just hugged his mom. They were talking at the same time, asking an array of questions. "Mom, are you okay? What happened? Are you sure you don't need to go to the hospital? Mary put her arms around the three of them, and then she became overwhelmed as tears ran down her face.

She loosened herself from their embraces, walked into the family room, and sat on the couch, with Monica on one side and Kermit sitting on the other side of her. Birdie and I were standing as she described how the accident had happened. I think talking about that experience helped Mary to put that emotional trauma behind her and overcome that frightening experience.

Mary was spared bodily harm. She would often say, "Willis, I know it was nothing but the grace of God that protected me that night!" A few days later, the insurance company declared the automobile a total loss. However, that accident did not deter Mary, as she was on the highway again the next week, driving to Ann Arbor. She persevered, driving rather it was in the rain, sleet, or snow those 136 miles round-trip three times a week.

Regardless of how long she had been commuting safely to and from the U of M, I still did not feel comfortable until I heard the garage door lift up, and I knew she was home safely. Some nights she would get home and flop down on the couch, stating, "baby, I had a long exhausting day." I would sit next to her and hug her. She would place her head on my chest, and her smile would appear. I knew she was not complaining but just stating that the circumstances she had encountered that day were a little fatiguing.

Mary's school year had rolled into 1982, and now she was in the home stretch. Periodically I would ask how her grades were overall. With the modesty she so eloquently displayed, she would hunch her shoulders up and down and say, "I'm doing okay. I think my grades are among the class leaders."

The year had passed fast, and we were approaching winter. It was now late November 1982, with Mary only having to complete her final examinations, and then her graduation was looming in front of her in late December. When Mary received the grades from her final exams, she was excited about driving the sixty-eight miles from Ann Arbor to home.

She came into the house with a big smile on her face and gave me an enthusiastic kiss. She said your inspiration worked very well, Willis Drake. What were your words about not accepting anything lower than a "C" grade? Well baby I got my final grades today, and I maintained an "A" average in my classes! I am graduating with "Cum Laude" honors.

I hugged Mary around her waist tightly and whispered in her ear, baby, I think you need some inspiration tonight. We both were cracking up as we were tightly embracing one another. Despite her overall school requirements and the job workload, Mary completed the semester with a high GPA (Grade Point Average) of "4.0."

Smiling from ear to ear, I congratulated Mary on her achievement and told her, "Baby, you choose any restaurant you want to have dinner to celebrate, and it will be just you and I having dinner together." She said, "I would like that."

There were only a few days that Mary had to attend activities in Ann Arbor prior to her graduation. In the meantime, she had time to shop for our family's Christmas presents. On top of Mary's pending graduation ceremony, the excitement of the holidays totally occupied her time.

Mary was upbeat all week. Christmas was two and a half weeks away, and Mary decided she wanted to go to dinner this Wednesday evening, and the two of us went to our favorite restaurant in Lakeview. This is the restaurant I would take Mary for dinner on our wedding anniversary day.

We had a 6:00 pm reservation on Wednesday, and entering the restaurant, Mary knew exactly what she wanted to order. The receptionist promptly seated us at five fifty-five pm in our favorite booth, sitting across from one another. The waiter was at our booth immediately, asking if we were ready to order. He gave us a dinner menu, but Mary only glanced at the menu, and she ordered her favorite steak dinner with baked potatoes and a side toss salad.

Then she whispered to the waiter, "be sure and save a slice of German Chocolate cake for my dessert." The waiter smiled and acknowledged he understood and assured Mary that he would.

The overall ambiance in the restaurant was enticing, which increased the satisfaction of enjoying good-tasting food. Mary said, "I need this evening to relax. After my busy schedule this year, and my graduation ceremony around the corner, I just now need to wound down mentally.

Willis, it was not the easiest thing to get through this year, but with your and the kid's help, I did well in my classes. Baby, I must admit that I am proud of the "Cum Laude" honor I earned."

It seemed like only minutes before the waiter appeared to serve our meal, and that was the only thing that stopped Mary from talking. The aroma from her steak dinner changed her train of thought, and she said baby, I am ready to eat. We blessed our food, and silence existed for several minutes as we dug in and enjoyed our meal.

The waiter returned and asked how everything was and if we needed anything else. Mary asked the waiter to put her German chocolate cake in a to-go bag. Looking at me with joy in her eyes, she said, "Willis, I really enjoyed my food, but I am too full to eat dessert now."

I paid the check and gave the waiter an extra-nice tip, and it was 6:55 pm when we left the restaurant. Driving home, Mary had her head on my shoulder, and she was floating on a natural high.

We arrived home feeling really good. Monica, with that curious smile on her face, said, "momma did you enjoy yourself having a night out with daddy?" Mary was smiling ear-to-ear and said, "Monica, I really enjoyed dinner, and it was so relaxing, and the food was really delicious. I had one of the best steaks that I have eaten in a while. Girl, your dad still knows how to treat me. He makes me feel incredibly special, which is why I love him." Monica was grinning and teasing her mom, "you still got what it takes for dad."

Mary was laughing as she walked back to our bedroom. Monica said, "Momma, you deserve to relax after earning your college degree. I am excited to see you walk across the stage next week to receive your degree.

I was in the bedroom when Mary walked in. She asked me to help unzip her dress, so she could lie down and relax. "Babe, be careful not to perpetuate the stereotypical idea that you will go to sleep after you eat." Now laughing, Mary responded, "I do not want to go to sleep; I just want to relax a little bit. Come lay down and relax with me so we can finish talking.

I flopped down next to Mary, lying on top of the bed covers. I do not know if it was by design on her part or if it was a spontaneous, intuitive action. However, Mary was now resting her head on my chest, relaxing, and she continued talking.

Quickly, she changed the subject saying, "Willis, with my head on your chest, I can hear your heartbeat so clearly. It's in these moments that I know, no matter what, everything will be all right." I was smiling and thought Mary's comment was a little hyperbole, but it did stroke my ego a bit. It felt personally stimulating to hear Mary declare confidence in me and believe that whatever her situation was, I would always "make it" okay.

The days rolled by quickly, and suddenly December 20th was here. Now the family was getting in the car to travel on I-94 to Ann Arbor. This was the route that Mary had traveled so many days to reach this pinnacle. That now had culminated in her graduating from the U of M. I felt immense gratitude for being able to attend Mary's graduation ceremony on Monday, December 20, 1982. I felt immensely proud when Mary walked across the stage and received her Bachelor of Science in Nursing (BSN) degree.

Birdie, Monica, Kermit, and I did not have the greatest vantage point to observe Mary receiving her degree, but it allowed us to express ourselves enthusiastically and with pride for her achievement as she walked across the stage and received her degree.

When the graduation ceremony was over, we rushed to the area where the graduates had assembled to meet their family members. When we arrived at the reception, Mary was beaming with pride as she hugged me, Birdie, Monica, and Kermit. Her eyes were moist, but no tears appeared.

We accompanied Mary to her nurses' reception; she only wanted to stay a few minutes. So we mingled at the reception, and Mary introduced Birdie, Monica, Kermit, and me to a few of her classmates. She sought out three younger classmates; she particularly wanted us to meet. As we approached them, they called her name and hugged and congratulated Mary. The young classmates seemed to admire Mary as their mature (mentor) classmate.

Joan Kohn, Mary's VA coworker, also graduated from the class, and we extended our congratulations to her as well. I believe Joan was a few years older than Mary. Periodically, the two would share a ride to class together; sometimes, they would study together.

Mary also, with tremendous zeal, introduced us to her mentor. It was satisfying for me to meet her, as Mary, throughout the year, had extolled her mentor; she is the only African-American professor I have met in the nursing program at the U of M. The kids and I shook hands with Mary's mentor; in kind, her mentor spoke very favorably of

Mary's accomplishments in the bachelor nursing program. As we were leaving, her mentor mentioned, "Mary, I want you to think about what I suggested."

We were near the exit door when Mary said, wait here a minute for me; I'm going to say bye to a few classmates I had not congratulated. It will only take me a minute, and she rushed off quickly.

I proudly focused my eyes on Mary as she congratulated her classmates and finished saying her goodbyes to them. As I observed Mary, I reflected on that day when I asked Mary's parents for their permission to marry her. I promised her parents that I would do everything possible for Mary to finish nursing school. Now Mary has her BSN degree from the University of Michigan, and I am so incredibly proud of her. She was "Destined and Determined" to be a nurse!

Driving home, Mary turned and looked at Birdie, Monica, and Kermit in the back seat of the car. Smiling, she said I love you'll.

Mary Pursues Her Master of Science (MSN) Degree
Mary's next milestone started in the Winter Semester of 1983 at the U of M Ann Arbor, and her goal was to obtain her Master of Science (MSN) degree. Working full-time at the VA, she had completed her BSN degree, and she realized that her MSN degree would be more difficult.

Mary got her ducks in a row when she decided to enroll for her MSN degree. She knew undertaking this course of action would require her total dedication to schooling. Therefore she requested to work on weekends only, two days a week, to maintain her civil-service status at the VA Hospital.

Mary was still in a state of euphoria the week following her graduation. This particular evening we were having a typical normal conversation. Mary had cuddled up to me; historically, this was her approach when she wanted to entice me to do something she wanted. Invariably she would cuddle and rest her head on my chest.

She would unbutton the top two buttons on my shirt and playfully pull the hair on my chest. So when this maneuver occurred, I always knew she had an ulterior motive. I played along with her approach because I enjoyed her attention and all the ego-stroking she gave me.

I responded by gently stroking Mary's face and asking in a soft voice what do you want me to do? I know you have something on your mind when you start pulling my chest hair. Raising her head from my chest and with a big smile on her face, she said, "I just like to pull the hair on your chest. However, you may think I have a secondary motive in mind, but I like pulling the hair on your chest.

Willis, I introduced you to my mentor, the African-American professor, at the graduation reception. She suggested that since I had done so well in the BSN nursing program, I should consider enrolling immediately in the master's nursing (MSN) program this semester. She specifically held a space open for me in the MSN degree program. Baby, it is a two-year program, and I think it would be to my advantage to continue straight through for the next two years and earn my MSN degree now.

I know it will not be a burden for you, but will it be too much of a strain on you and the family if I continue with school and get my master's degree now? I will still have to drive to Ann Arbor three, or more times a week. The VA personnel office approved me working part-time on the weekend; they also confirmed that I would maintain my nursing position and civil service status."

I assured Mary, "We as a family will continue doing whatever it takes for you to get your master's degree. Is all this affectionate attention you are delving out now, what this is about, girl?" Mary put her arms around my neck and gave me a passionate kiss. Then she said, "Willis, thanks for your support, and I love you man." With that decision made, Mary continued the next semester at the U of M, working towards her master's (MSN) degree.

Neither Mary nor I had the spiritual acumen to pray for these job-related situations or conditions. However, every condition identified above was necessary for Mary to earn her MSN Degree. Having those conditions granted were tantamount to Mary being successful in college.

Every step Mary had taken was falling into place. We were particularly in sound financial shape. Our house was paid off, and Mary working part-time would not be a problem financially. We would continue to save Mary's income.

Like most things that require arduous work and determination, there is always a bump in the road. However, nothing monumental got in Mary's path on the way to earning her Master's degree.

Mary again would drive 136 miles round-trip to Ann Arbor, at least three days a week and sometimes more. This had become her modus operandi over the past several years, and she was versed in the traffic patterns, going to, and coming from Ann Arbor. Her home and work schedules were conducive to the study habits required to earn her Master's degree.

Mary had many late-night study sessions at the kitchen table of our home. She said the master's program was very demanding, and it required her consistent detail attention. However, she said, "from the beginning in this one class, the professor did not care for me without provocation. We never established the best rapport between us as a student and instructor."

On several occasions, Mary would come home frustrated, and she would vent to me, explaining that her class instructor (professor) seemed intimidated by her relationship with the young students in the class. Particularly when she asked the instructor a question in front of the class, Mary thought the professor may have considered her question a challenge to her "subject matter knowledge."

Mary was a mature intelligent registered nurse in her early forties, and many of her young student classmates sought her advice. Mary surmised that the instructor resented her leadership and acceptability among the young students.

At the end of the semester, this particular evening, Mary was furious when she got home from class. She stormed into the house, and she was obviously highly agitated. It was so out of character for her to display that type of attitude. I tried greeting her normally, but she was livid for some reason, unbeknownst to me.

She said hi, baby, and then immediately sat down at the kitchen table. She rested her head in both hands; and said I am just a little upset. How are you, Willis? I moved closer and put my hand on her head; are you okay, babe? What's going on?

She raised her head and looked at me. Willis, I can't believe this one instructor gave me a "C minus" (C-) grade for the course. Mary said, I worked my tail off, and based on my class papers and test grades, I earned at least a B grade in that class.

She rose from the chair and walked to the family room. Standing in front of the TV, she said Willis, I discussed my grade with my instructor, but she would not consider my point of view. Neither would she accept the objective facts supporting my higher grade in the class. I will discuss this issue with my mentor when I return to school next week.

Mary cooled down some as we finished talking during the night. She planned to talk with her mentor, whom she highly respected. When Mary returned to school, she discussed the situation with her mentor, who agreed with Mary's position. However, she explained to Mary that "you are in the first year of the master's program. You might win this battle, but you could lose the war. So you need to evaluate if it is worth elevating "your grade issue" to a higher level." Mary decided not to appeal her grade discrepancy.

Mary overcame the issues with that one instructor and now has completed her college nursing MSN program. On May 3, 1985, we were back at " Michigan University" watching Mary take her final steps across the stage and graciously receive her "**Master of Science (psychiatric-Mental Health Nursing) MSN degree.**"

Unfortunately, when Mary completed her master's program, that C-grade prevented her from graduating with "Cum Laude" honors in the "Master of Science in Psychiatric-Mental Health Nursing. In every other class during the two years of her Master's program, Mary earned a grade of "A or B."

I observed as I proudly watched Mary walk across the stage to receive her MSN degree. I had a vivid image in my mind of her, the seventeen-year-old student nurse at the Homer G. nursing school.

My thoughts were reflective as the ensuing years unfolded; I was constantly by Mary's side encouraging, supporting, and motivating her to reach the goal of being a registered nurse. I was there in 1964 when she graduated from Homer G. hospital nursing school, following the birth of our two children, and I saw on December 20, 1982, the results of what determination and destiny would bring when she received her "Bachelor of Science in Nursing (BSN) degree." Again, on May 3, 1985, I witnessed when she received her Master of Science (psychiatric-Mental Health Nursing) MSN degree.

Mary has completed her college education with her BSN and MSN degrees. Over time, Mary and I discussed the feasibility of relocating from Battle Creek to Virginia if a job opportunity became available. The time was perfect when in April 1985, a position at HQs DLA became available, and Mary would graduate from the U of M a few weeks later in May 1985.

CHAPTER 35

Willis—Headquarters (HQ's) DLA In Virginia

A T THIS POINT, WE HAD lived in Springfield, Michigan, for eleven years. Now that Mary had finished college, the possibility of me accepting a job at Headquarters Defense Logistics Agency (HQs DLA) and relocating to Virginia grew exponentially.

For two years, HQs DLA management personnel "recruited me heavily to accept a position at DLA. After Mary graduated with her MSN (Master's in Science) Nursing Degree, a job opportunity became available for me to consider.

Cliff Noaiell, my former officemate at DLSC in 1983, had accepted a job at HQs DLA. Cliff and I talked several times a month, and he and his wife, Barbara, enjoyed living in the Virginia area.

Professionally, I had established a well-earned reputation as an exceptional program/project manager. Cliff and his supervisor Willard Smith, whom I knew well, encouraged their Division Chief, Hank Fillippi, to hire me for a job in the Standardization and Engineering Division at HQs DLA.

During one of our routine late-night conversations, Mary and I seriously discussed my accepting a job at HQs DLA. Mary said we only have

Kermit in high school. Birdie and Monica had spent two years in college, but neither was currently enrolled in college. So if the opportunity becomes available, you should apply and accept the job.

Within two months, a vacancy in the Cataloging Division at HQs DLA was advertised. Mary and I made the decision that I would apply for the job. I was selected and hired as a GS-13 Supply Cataloger, and we would move to Virginia. Mary was confident she could get a job at the Veteran Administration (VA) in Washington, DC.

Mary and I had close friends, Charles, (and Emma) Smith, who had transferred to HQs DLA a year ago. I had known Charles since our Sumner High School days in St. Louis. We knew other close friends, Sam Burge, Denise Hobson, Robert (Bob) Hobson, and Loretta Bowman, who worked at the Federal Center in Battle Creek and had transferred to the Alexandria, Virginia area. We had a cadre of friends and colleagues to connect and socialize within the area.

A coworker from Battle Creek, Tisa Cross, had transferred to the HQs Cataloging Division, working for Dean Erwin, the Cataloging Division Chief, who I also knew. I heard he was the person that had overridden his Branch Chief's selection for the job I had applied for, but Dean Erwin instead selected me for the job.

I reported to HQs DLA in mid-April 1985. Mary and the family remained in Springfield, Michigan, until Kermit's school year ended in June. I rented an apartment unit at the Oakwood Apartments in Alexandria, VA. It was located five minutes from Cameron Station Army Base, Alexandria, Virginia, where HQs DLA was located. Living in the apartment, I didn't have to contend with traffic issues getting to work.

I didn't seriously house hunt during the time I was living in the apartment by myself. Again I decided to defer buying a house until Mary could come and seriously look for a house she wanted to buy.

Our friends, Charles and Emma Smith, lived in Burke, Virginia, about 35 minutes from HQs DLA. On a few weekends, I would visit their home, kick back with Charles, shoot the breeze, and eat dinner with their family. Also, on a few occasions, I attended their son Dion's track meet when he was a student at Lake Braddock High School.

Before Kermit's school was out for the summer, in late May 1985, Mary took a week off from work and came to Alexandria to look for a house. I contacted two real estate agents, but neither gave me a comfortable feeling regarding finding a house we would consider buying. Mary looked at a few houses, but nothing seriously materialized.

We visited our friends Charles and Emma, who were buying a townhouse in Burke, VA. So we drove through the Burke area; Mary said she liked the homes and the area in general. However, we also looked at a few houses in Springfield and Fairfax, Virginia.

Mary was a little frustrated as she said that having only one week to find a house she would be totally satisfied with was insufficient time for her. However, she decided she wanted to live in the Burke, VA area, and she wanted a single-family house, not a townhouse.

We had not found a house yet to bring our family to live in Virginia, and Kermit's school would be out in a few weeks. Now the pressure was on me to find a house to rent that met Mary's requirements, "A single-family house in Burke, VA."

We knew once our family was relocated and living in Virginia, Mary could work with a realtor and take sufficient time to find the right house for us to buy. Also, becoming familiar with the general geographical area would allow her to have better knowledge to consider where to buy a house, possibly other than in Burke, VA.

In short order, I found a house to rent. I called Mary and described the house to her, and we agreed that I would rent the house. I had to sign a one-year lease, on the newly built three-year-old house, with four bedrooms and two and a half bathrooms. The house was located in a nice neighborhood in the Longwood Knolls Subdivision in Burke, VA.

Mary was tasked with supervising "packing up" our home possessions to move to Virginia. We hired a moving company to pack and box up everything in the house, put it on the moving van, transport everything to Virginia, and put the furniture and everything in our rented house.

When Mary, Monica, and Kermit Matthew arrived in Virginia that afternoon and saw the house and the community for the first time, they all were especially pleased, and Mary was delighted with the house. She said in many ways, the houses and the neighborhood reminded her of the Springfield, MI., area where we owned our house. By 7:00 pm that evening, the movers had completed putting the furniture in the house.

The next order of business was to get Kermit registered at the Lake Braddock High School. It was a few months before school would start, and the week we moved into the house, Kermit met Marcus Crockett, a teenager his age who lived in the neighborhood. Instantly, they became best friends and remained friends throughout their four years of high school and are still friends now.

There was never any pressure for Mary to work, so she decided to take time off and not work immediately. Additionally, by not working, she had the luxury of learning about the neighborhoods where we might want to buy a house.

Unfortunately, there was no "Mildred Wright" to assist Mary with information sharing regarding the new community we would be living in. However, we connected with friends from work, which suggested medical and other service professionals we would need services from. Loretta Bowman, who we knew from Battle Creek, got us associated with the church she was a member of; Alleyne AME Church, 1419 King St. Alexandria, VA 22314.

Also, as Mary became familiar with Virginia's geographical areas, she became more adventurous in looking at houses throughout the surrounding areas. Mary would often say, Willis, one day, I want you to buy me a brand-new constructed house that no one has owned or lived in. We would laugh, and I agreed that, possibly, one day, I would buy her a newly constructed house.

As time rolled along, fall turned into winter, and Mary was content with being a stay-at-home mom and wife. Our daughter Monica, who had moved to Virginia with us, had informed us in November that her "boyfriend, Gordon Zinn," was coming to visit her for the Thanksgiving holiday weekend, and he wanted to talk to me.

It was Thanksgiving Day when Gordon came to ask for my permission to marry Monica. Mary was highly upset with Monica because she had not given us any indication that she and Gordon were planning to get married. We gave them our blessings to get married, and Gordon gave Monica an engagement ring that day. They got married the following month, on December 14, 1985.

Mary had to quickly arrange for a home wedding and reception at the house. Monica and Gordon returned to Battle Creek, Michigan, to live. The following spring of 1986, Monica and Gordon traveled to St. Louis so she could introduce her husband to her grandparents and family.

During their visit to St. Louis, Mary arranged for a reception to formally present Monica and her husband, Gordon, to our family members in the East St. Louis and St. Louis areas. Gordon, with his personality, was readily welcomed by both sides of our families. He also received official acknowledgment from my mother that he would be a good husband to Monica. My mother's words rang true, as Monica and Gordon were married for 29 years until he passed on February 5, 2014.

Gordon was a wonderful husband to Monica and a terrific father to their only child Adriana, who was born on June 29, 1993. Moreover, Gordon was more like a son than a son-in-law to Mary and me.

CHAPTER 36

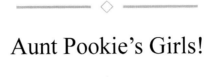

Aunt Pookie's Girls!

I HAD OFTEN WONDERED WHAT MOTIVATED Mary to be so benevolent to the next generation of her family. Perhaps, it was a carryover from her big sister's role growing up watching out for her younger siblings. Maybe it was remembering the love, care, and attention she received from her aunts, being the only girl in the family for many years. Collectively these traits may have helped shape and mold Mary's caring spirit.

However, more than anything, likely her generosity in giving back was the example her mother provided through her actions when she babysat Willis Jr. (Birdie), which allowed Mary to finish nursing school and become a registered nurse.

Now regardless of the reason, at this point in her life, Mary had reaped the benefit of being a wonderful mother, a terrific wife, and having a husband that loved her. She also had a successful professional nursing career behind her as a dedicated and accomplished Registered Nurse (RN).

Within her final year of working, she was on the cusp of retiring, and her retirement plan was on point. Upon retiring in April 2004, she would step immediately into her active role as the MDI (Male Duck Inc.) Secretary-Treasurer and Office Manager. Although she was still working, she would work from home and set her own work schedule, hours, and the amount of time she worked.

It's vague in my memory if Mary discussed with me, prior to her retirement, her plan to embark on her benevolent activities in 2003. During our normal daily conversations, our granddaughter, Adriana, constantly crept into our routine conversation. She was getting older and would be a teenager soon. As a normal progression, inherently as a teenager, she would likely not want to share her summers with her grandparents often.

Mary's kind and loving heart is one reason I was drawn to her initially. The impulse and motivation that penetrated Mary's thoughts to become a mentor and an active supporter for her granddaughter and great nieces' future seemed spontaneous. I am not certain if it was innate or a quality she acquired from her many wonderful life experiences. Regardless, her actions were to give back and promote her young female family members.

Early in our marriage, Willis Jr. and Monica were maybe 4 or 5 years old after Mary finished nursing school. When Mary's sisters and brothers were young kids, we often took them on various fun summer outings with my nieces and nephews.

It may have been something routine as going to the St. Louis zoo, Chain of Rocks Amusement Park, drive-in movies, and any event that would be fun for them. A summer highlight was also going to the **Teamsters** Local 688 facility in **Pevely**, Missouri. Our financial resources were the only restrictions that prohibited the activities to which we could expose the kids.

As is often the case, time seems to accelerate faster when you are thirty years old. Suddenly, Mary's brother David was a young adult and now had children, A'Ryanne and Dierdre (Dee Dee). Her nieces looked up very highly to Mary, their "Aunt Pookie."

Our oldest children, Willis Jr. (Birdie) and Monica, were a generation older than David's children and their brother Kermit. However, Kermit was the oldest in the generational age group of his cousins, A'Ryanne

Byas, Dierdre (Dee Dee) Byas-Rodgers, and Terez Ivy. Mary's brother Terry and her sister Margaret Ann, their first child, was born approximately five years later.

Mary and I had already embraced our role of aunt and uncle on my side of our family. Now for Mary's side of our family, she was "Aunt Pookie," and I was "Uncle Willis." When we visited East St. Louis on vacation, Mary established a terrific aunt and niece relationship with A'Ryanne and Dee Dee. Their relationship matured as the girls became teenagers. Mary often encouraged her nieces to go to college, and she was excited when Dee Dee went off to college.

Now the cycle of life was continuing, as Mary's nieces, A'Ryanne and Dee Dee, had children now. Along with this next generation of great-nieces was the commingling, age-wise, of Mary's siblings Terry's (Terrence Jr., Cedric, Terrianna, and Keyarra) and Margaret Ann's son (Jason) children. With us being older now, Mary's maternal instincts kicked in, and her desire to nurture the younger generations in our collective family increased.

Mary's relationship as an aunt with her great nieces allowed her a position of influence on the next generation of family members. Particularly, she fostered a special mentoring relationship with her granddaughter, Adriana Drake Zinn-Mark, as well as her nieces, Terrianna Byas-Jackson, Keyarra Byas, and Stephanie Wooten, who were basically the same age; as-well-as her great-nieces Amber Rodgers, Erin Rodgers, and Cicily Byas.

Mary wanted to take Adriana and her niece and great-nieces' on a getaway vacation this summer. She wanted to expose them to fun experiences that would enhance their horizons and increase their expectations for their future. Similarly, to a lesser extent, she had done this with her young sisters Mona and Margaret Ann when they were growing up.

She wanted her nieces, great-nieces, and granddaughter exposed to that same type of motivation and inspiration also. Her idea was to take the girls on an in-state excursion, so they could experience something different and more than what their neighborhood surroundings uniquely provided.

Periodically, Mary would share her thoughts with me regarding where she wanted to take the girls on vacation. I think she primarily wanted me to listen, more so than for my input. On this particular day, she was standing in the middle of the kitchen with her right hand on her waist and her left hand on her chin. It was a pose that represented deep thought.

Then unexpectedly, like a bolt of lightning, she said, "Willis, I believe it was in the summer of 1967 when you took me to the Lake of the Ozarks and sister Shirley and Stan; Marvin and Vickie went with us.

I have checked out both the Ozarks and the Branson areas. I want to take "the girls" to Branson, Missouri, where we can use our MDI timeshare exchange privileges for our lodging accommodations. There are many fun outdoor activities, live entertainment, museums, bumper cars, boat rides, and a spa that I am sure the girls will enjoy.

They will be exposed to an environment that's different from the city's landscape of brick and mortar where they live. I want them to splash around in the lake or the resort's swimming pool. Just enjoy the amusement activities, and they can have fun participating in a totally different environment.

Listening to Mary talk, I was impressed! I remember when we were much younger and without the financial resources that we now have, how we would take the kids, including our nieces and nephews, to the amusement parks and baseball games, at our expense.

I asked Mary what I could do to help her with this adventure. Smiling, she said, "Baby, I am going to ask Mona and Margaret Ann to help chaperone the girls on this trip. At my age, I don't have the energy to keep up with these energetic young girls."

From that point, Mary continued with her plans to take "the girls" to Branson, Missouri. It would be a four-day excursion, and she had to make two separate lodging reservations to accommodate the total of four days. One reservation for the first night was at the Fairfield Mountain Vista, and a second was at the Fairfield Branson at the Falls for the remaining three nights of the trip.

I stayed in St. Louis as Mary and "Aunt Pookie's Girls" departed on their excursion to Branson, Missouri. This trip occurred at the last of July and the beginning of August 2003. The girls were nine to eleven years old. They were at an impressionable age and would soon enter junior high school.

At this point in our lives, Mary and I had traveled to many states in the United States. She was comfortable traveling on the highways, and with her sisters also being experienced highway drivers, she was comfortable making the trip without me. Mary financed the trip using the discretionary income she had available. She did not ask me for any financial support for the trip. She funded the entire trip, which included all the transportation, lodging, entertainment, food, and souvenir expenses.

This was, in effect, a "trial balloon" of sorts. Depending on the outcome of this trip, it would be the foundation for Mary planning future trips for "the girls." Mary envisioned staying connected to the girls as they matured through high school and into college. On this first vacation trip, the girls, Terrianna and Keyarra Byas, Amber, Erin Rogers, Cicily Byas, Stephanie Wooten, and Adriana Zinn, were going to spend four days over the weekend together.

Mary was planting a seed of possibility in the minds of "Aunt Pookie's girls." Besides the girls having fun, her primary objective was to motivate them and have them aspire to get a college education. She wanted the girls to be equipped to create a better life for themselves in the future.

Mary was delighted to expose "Aunt Pookie's girls" to a world of possibilities outside their regular East St. Louis environment. Experiences like this could inspire them to believe that all dreams are possible. Even more so, with hard work, a college education, and the grace of God, anything is possible.

Moreover, the trip would provide "the girls" with the experience of staying in a resort-style vacation facility with exceptional accommodations and all the amenities and comforts they needed. They would enjoy good food and also some "junk" food too. Plus enjoy different entertainment and amusement activities that would provide them exceptional fun.

Mary observed, as the week wound down, that each girl had chronicled on paper (and in their mind and heart) their personal experiences that would be locked in their memory forever. Mary was hopeful that this experience would be a motivator for their future. There were fun, temper tantrums, pouting, and a memorable experience that 9, 10, and 11-year-old girls would never forget.

It was remarkable that each of "Aunt Pookie's girls" presented her with handwritten or typed chronicled experiences as an expression of thanking her for a marvelous vacation. I was not able to include those documents in this book, but Mary cherished and preserved them.

Arriving home from Branson and returning to East St. Louis, Mary emerged from the car, and we excitedly greeted one another. Immediately I discerned that she was a little fatigued. As the mothers welcomed their girls home, it was rewarding to see the parents hugging and pampering their children, asking if they had enjoyed themselves and had fun.

Mary said her goodbyes to the girls, and we drove back to St. Louis to the hotel. Mary said they had a wonderful time. A smile caressed her face, and she said as they were driving back home, the girls said "they were going to write about their experience of this weekend, so they could look back on it in later years.

Later, Mary confided that "she could have used my help on the trip." However, she wanted the trip to be primarily a "girls-only" experience. The only boy on the trip was Mary's seven years old great-nephew Brendon Byas. By interacting with her nieces, Mary got to know the young girls' personalities. It was amazing to hear how similar and yet different the cousins were.

Mary and I prepared to return to Burke, Virginia, in a few days. Now returning home, it was comical to me; however, in advance, Mary was soliciting my help for when she would take "the girls" on their next trip. In a humble voice, she said, "Willis, the next trip that I take the girls on will probably be next year. I want you to go with me on that trip, okay."

In a lighthearted way, I started laughing. "Baby, you just can't stand to be away from me for one week, can you?" Mary was smiling as she stated matter of fact, "Willis, don't flatter yourself, man. It's purely a management and planning issue, but I do like having you close by me.

Man, you constantly remind me that you are the "master planner." So I need your help to plan and coordinate the activities for the girls' next trip. Laughing, I agreed, "Okay, I will go on the next trip with you and the girls."

Periodically, during the year, Mary stayed in contact with "the girls" directly or indirectly through their parents. She frequently interacted with her granddaughter Adriana, who lived in Sagamore Hills, Ohio. She also stayed in contact with her sisters, Mona and Margaret Ann; that was her "grapevine" to keep up with how "the girls" were doing.

Unbeknownst to me, as the idea marinated in her mind in the spring of 2004, Mary first broached with me her idea of taking "the girls" on vacation to Chicago this summer. It was a Saturday morning, and Mary and I were talking at the kitchen table. She asked nonchalantly, "Willis, how far is St. Louis from Chicago? Quizzically looking at her, "I don't know how many miles it is, but it will take five or six hours to drive from St. Louis to Chicago."

Gazing wide-eyed into space, Mary said, "if we drove from St. Louis to Chicago, we would first need to rent two minivans. Then we would need someone to drive the vans; and a backup driver for each van. We would have to travel caravan style, with the vans trailing one another. I know that it could be unsafe to drive on the highway. With her attention focused on me, she said, "Willis, what are your thoughts on driving from St. Louis to Chicago for the girl's vacation this year?

While Mary was talking, I was observing her face. I could see that her thought process was in high gear. She said, "for this trip; I want "my girls" to fly on an airplane. It would be the first experience flying for most of them." So just like that, Mary made a decision to travel to Chicago by airplane.

Everything in Mary's plan materialized one month before the trip was scheduled. When summer rolled around, Mary had made all the necessary arrangements for the trip. We were in St. Louis on the day of travel. With their suitcases packed, "Aunt Pookie's girls" piled into the cars, going to St. Louis Lambert Airport.

Naturally, the girls were extremely excited, anticipating their maiden airplane flight. Seeing their faces, it was only happiness, no fear of getting ready to fly from St. Louis to Chicago. As the girls were boarding the plane, the joy extended into sheer jubilance, and they were asked to settle down a little.

It was a small American Eagle airplane, and Mary had pre-determined the girls seating arrangements. Suddenly, Erin was upset, crying, and wanted to sit next to her big sister Amber. Mary made that seating adjustment, and now the laughter and chatter among the girls resumed.

The airplane roared down the runway. As the plane ascended in the air, looking at "the girls," there was a collection of awe, slight fear, amazement, and total exhilaration. The airplane was now flying above the clouds, and seeing the expression on each girl's face, was a memory to behold. Their joy was something I will always remember.

The flight technically was short; flying from St. Louis to Chicago would only take one hour and 15 minutes. As the airplane's wheels touched down on the runway at O'Hare's airport, the girls made, oh and ah, sounds as the airplane bounced slightly. Taking their backpacks from the overhead compartments, they got off the airplane with the same exuberance when they boarded the plane.

The girls were saying to each other how they felt flying on an airplane. It was sort of predictable, based on a few of the girls' personalities. That a comment stating, "I was afraid the plane was going to fall out of the sky," was inevitable. That comment evocated the usual response, "girl, you are so crazy," followed by laughter.

With Mona, Margaret Ann, and Mary, we conveniently picked up the rental cars and got registered in the hotel. We stayed at a nice hotel. The itinerary for the vacation included visiting several Chicago Museums and going to the waterfront, where there were interesting and fun activities for the girls to participate in. Mary again funded the complete cost of the entire trip.

This was the second year Mary arranged for "the girls" to have a new life experience. Her example of exposing the next generation of young girls in their families to new experiences has evolved. Mary built a solid foundation as an example to motivate and inspire the young girls in her family. Several of her cousins from East St. Louis drove their daughters to Chicago to join "Aunt Pookie's girls."

In our family, there is an expression that says, "Invest your time in children when they are young, and you will have an influence on them when they are older." Soon Mary's young nieces became teenagers, and they entered high school. She, along with their parents, emphasized the need for them to do well in school, so they would be prepared to attend college.

Mary invested her time and other resources to help prepare and motivate her granddaughter, nieces, and great-nieces to get a college education. To date, five of the seven "Aunt Pookie's girls" have earned their college bachelor's degree, and two are pursuing their master's degree. One niece, Stephanie Wooten, has earned her master's degree and is attending Southern Illinois University (SIU) Medical School.

On December 15, 2022, I received a text message from Stephanie, inviting me to her graduation from medical school on May 20, 2023. She will graduate as a medical doctor in her specialty of pediatrics. I immediately made my airline reservation, so I will be among the family members applauding Stephanie as she walks across the stage to receive her medical degree. I also know that her "Aunt Pookie" will be looking down smiling on one of her girls, acknowledging a job very well done Stephanie!

Moreover, Mary is a testament that it is never too late to earn a college degree. She had been married for sixteen years when she entered college to get her Bachelor of Science in Nursing degree, and she graduated in December 1982 when she was forty-one years old.

Aunt Pookie's girls, who have earned their degrees, and those without college degrees, have jobs and can support themselves independently. That was "Aunt Pookie's" (Mary's) goal for her girls.

However, Aunt Pookie had a cadre of nephews that were as endearing to her as well. Not only did we provide exposure on outings for entertainment to a lesser extent to the nephews; but we as Aunt Pookie and Uncle Willis, show them our encouragement to do as well as they could in their lives as well.

Mary's nephew Terez Ivy after finishing college did not have the best job opportunities available to him career wise, in the East St. Louis area. He moved to Virginia and lived with his Aunt Pookie and Uncle Willis, as part of our family. He was able to get established in the computer technology area career wise, he purchased a home and created a small business. Aunt Pookie and Uncle Willis had a positive influence on Terez's life.

CHAPTER 37

Mary—Washington DC, VA Hospital

MARY HAD DECIDED TO TAKE a break, time off, from working prior to moving to Virginia. So she resigned from her position at the Battle Creek VA instead of transferring to the U.S. Department of Veterans Affairs—Washington DC VA Medical Center. Therefore, technically she would have to apply for an RN position at the Washington DC Veterans Administration (VA) Medical Center, the same as any person seeking employment would.

Mary did not work outside the home for seven months after we moved to Virginia. Shortly after the New Year 1986, she announced to Kermit and me that she decided to go back to work. Kermit's response was a causal "okay, mom," like you would expect from a typical 16-year-old teenager.

I made a comical remark: "I had gotten used to coming home to well-cooked meals for dinner." Mary laughed, and her retort had its comical tone. Smiling, she said, "baby, I know you can burn in the kitchen very well yourself, and it hasn't been that long ago either. So don't try and flatter me with this "well-cooked meals for dinner scenario." We all laughed, and Kermit injected his humor, commenting, "Momma, I must say that your cooking does taste better than dad's cooking."

We had a good laugh, and in a more serious tone now, Mary said, "I believe, having worked for the VA Hospital in Battle Creek, I will be hired at the Washington DC, VA Medical Center."

Mary certainly wasn't "clairvoyant," but her job application and review process was expedited, and she was hired expeditiously. Within two weeks after her job interview, she started working for the Washington DC VA at 50 Irving St. NW, Washington, DC 20422.

Mary worked the morning shift from 8:00 am to 4:30 pm. However, during the first few days driving to work, she immediately understood the rush hour traffic I had alluded to earlier, which was much worse than the St. Louis rush hour traffic. I can now genuinely appreciate the 15 minutes commute to work in Battle Creek.

When Mary got home from work that first day, she was exasperated by her commute experience. Willis, living in Virginia for seven months, I experienced some heavy traffic during the middle of the day. However, I had no idea how horrific the commute rush hour traffic was from Virginia to the District (DC). Baby, sitting in traffic for hours to get to work is overwhelming, and getting home from work in the evenings is more of a headache.

During my job orientation walkthrough, I realized I would have more latitude to institute new nursing concepts. I think having more flexibility and autonomy to perform my job here at the DC VA Center will be a plus professionally for me.

The programs at the DC VA Center are more in line with the ideals I have in mind; and what I learned through my master's education program. I will have an opportunity to use my ingenuity and knowledge to establish programs I initiate to assist my VA patients.

Despite the traffic issue, Mary left each morning to go to work enthusiastically to her job. In the evenings, she would describe her coworkers as she was learning their personalities. In short order, she had emerged by the end of the month, being accepted very well into the current DC

VA nursing culture. Moreover, Mary's primary concern and interest were her VA patients and how she could improve their lives.

Periodically Mary worked the night shift, where the traffic was not as stressful getting to and from work. However, it required me to stay up past midnight to ensure Mary was home safely.

Mary went to work every day with her agenda wanting to help her patients, particularly the female veterans that had suffered sexual abuse in the military. With her professionalism, nursing knowledge, and hard work ethic, her patients trusted her.

As a rule, neither Mary nor I would bring our problems from the job home. As we would tell one another, we would shake off the dust from work when we crossed the threshold of our home in the evening. However, in certain situations, we had certain job-related conversations that required Mary to be consoled, and only a husband could provide.

Mary would need my ear to extricate some of the sad stories that her female patients had shared with her. She was a strong advocate for getting women's help, and it was rewarding for her when she saw a woman overcome some of her mental, emotional, and psychological problems as a result of her military service.

During those few times that Mary required me to just hold her tightly and listen and console her regarding a situation a patient had shared with her, that was so painful. Mary just needed to know how much I loved her. She would tell me, "Willis, you remember I mentioned "Ms. Doe" that I was working with to get help to function more independently on her own? I saw her today, and we talked; she is doing very well.

She said she could use some clothes to expand her professional wardrobe, to wear to the job that she now has. She and I are about the same size, and I will give her some appropriate casual work outfits that I know will enhance her wardrobe for work.

There were comparable stories, both male and female, that Mary had shared with me over the years she worked at the DC VA Hospital. I would tease Mary to lighten the atmosphere when she was conveying her emotional experiences with her patients. Sometimes Mary would give her patients a few dollars "gift loan," as she would call it.

I often extolled Mary for being "Destined and Determined to be a nurse." I would tell her how proud I was of her and how her caring for her patients was admirable and spiritually right. Then I would flirt with her and tell her I could use a little attention myself. Mary would laugh and say, "Willis, you never have a problem in that area. Now, do you? You always get my attention, any time, or all the time, baby. I love you, man."

Mary Establishes a Self-Sustained Program for Veterans at the VA
Over time working at the DC VA, there was one program, the Partial Hospitalization Program (PHP), that Mary established, and she was enormously proud of its success. This was an outpatient mental health program. Mary fostered and initiated the PHP program for the VA hospitalized resident patients that were able to be transitioned from being resident patients in the VA hospital to becoming functional persons living independently or semi-independent in an apartment or house on their own.

The Department of Veterans Affairs presented "Mary Drake, RN" a Certificate of Appreciation, and the words on the certificate were as follows: The veterans of the PHP program have expressed their appreciation for the outstanding educational, spiritual, and professional guidance that they receive from you on a daily basis. They have said that the PHP program has enabled them to re-establish their focus on life and has helped improve their family and overall social lives. The Medical Center Director, Sanford M. Garfunkel, said, "I add my thanks to those you serve. Thank you for a job well done."

One of Mary's coworkers in this PHP program was Mr. Percy Norman. He was a young man that Mary was proud of, and she often commented to me about him and his young family. She referred to him as one of her "kids." We periodically associated with Percy and his wife and participated in some milestones in their family lives, including celebrating their daughter's first birthday.

Mary also enjoyed working with Carol Ward, whom she considered a good friend. The workforce at the VA, on the unit where Mary was assigned, was a close-knit group working under their head nurse, Felion Hankerson. Mary and I attended the social gatherings and parties that the nursing staff sponsored. Notably, during the Christmas holidays, the staff on Mary's unit would have a gathering and share their ethnic foods and have a wonderful time together.

CHAPTER 38

⸻ ◇ ⸻

Retirement from the VA, 2004

⸻ ◇ ⸻

MARY HAD GONE THROUGH ANOTHER winter commuting to and from work in the District of Columbia. The weather had changed, and the temperature was warmer as March roared to a mild end. Now April was on the home front, and Mary had only two weeks left on the job before her retirement.

Every evening when Mary got home, she appeared to be in somewhat of a pensive mood. During the last week on the job, she showed signs of some anxiety and uneasiness but not discontent. Silently I began to wonder if Mary had second thoughts about her retirement. Having retired three years earlier, I could relate to the feelings she was experiencing, nervousness and uncertainty.

On Tuesday evening, when she got home, I heard the garage door open as usual. It only took Mary a few seconds to open the door and walk into the house. She was carrying a small box, and she put it on the chair in the family room.

She said hey babe, how are you; as she closed the door and went to hang up her coat in the hall closet. I was sitting on the couch in the family room watching TV. Taking my eyes off the TV for a moment, I glanced up at her; and said, "hi, I am fine; how was your day?"

Walking slowly, she came and flopped down on the couch next to me. Smiling, she hunched her shoulders up and down and said, "oh, I guess it was a so-so day. I spent most of the day clearing my desk and personal items in the office. Pointing to the box on the chair, see the box I brought home. It has a few personal mementos from over the 18 years I have worked at the Washington DC VA center.

I scooted closer to Mary, pulled her towards me, and hugged her. That gesture generated a smile on her face, and she said, "baby can you imagine I will be fully retired from the VA shortly? I am feeling a little nostalgic, as I only have a few more days to work, but I have genuinely enjoyed my nursing career. The news on the TV was signing off, and I asked Mary if she was ready to eat.

We both rose from the couch, and Mary went to set the table, and I heated the food in the microwave. With just the two of us sitting at the dinner table eating dinner, we had a conversation mostly about Mary being retired in a few days.

Friday morning, before leaving for work, Mary said babe, this is it. She had a smile on her face, and I knew she had mixed emotions, as anyone would have, who dedicated so much of their lives to caring for others. I walked her to the door leading into the garage, I gave her a tight hug, and she kissed me goodbye.

Observing Mary going to her job for the last day was sort of strange. She had "energy in her step" as she slid behind the steering wheel of her car. Now with excitement in her voice, she said loudly, "Willis, can you believe it? Today is the last day I will be driving down I-95 to the VA Medical Center.

Laughing joyfully, she backed the car out of the garage and went down the driveway, heading to work at the VA for the last time. I closed the garage door, and I thought Mary had spent close to 40 years as a nurse in two states, Missouri and Michigan, and in the Washington District of Columbia, the capital of the United States.

Now her day was over, and returning home on April 2, 2004, Mary Ann Byas-Drake was retired from the U.S. Department of Veterans Affairs—"Veteran Administration (VA)." She had completed twenty-five years of dedicated nursing services at the VA Hospital system.

Around the usual time, I heard the garage door open that evening when Mary got home. She walked into the family room, greeted me as usual, and closed the door behind her. She was hanging up her coat in the hall closet, and this routine would now cease.

With a smile on her face, from ear to ear, she said, babe, I am officially retired from the VA. As she was hanging up her coat, I walked from the kitchen. I put my arms around her waist, hugged her tightly, kissed her, and told her, "baby, you had a wonderful career that you should be enormously proud of.

I could see Mary's emotional feelings were creeping in at the moment. "Mary, just think back over your career when you were able to help young teenage girls, to the point where now you are caring for and counseling military veterans that were confused in the present and not certain what was in store for them the next day.

Mary said, "I feel particularly good about my nursing career, and I know that I was a positive influence on patients I encountered throughout my professional nursing career." That is a statement that Mary Ann Byas-Drake made to close the chapter on her nursing career.

Our routine when Mary arrived home that evening did not waver. She said, "I am hungry," and we sat down at the table, and I blessed the food, and we ate dinner and talked. That smile on Mary's face was still illuminating, and she said, "today, before I left work, I was sitting in my office, and I reflected on my nursing career.

Willis, my first thought was, and I honestly believe this. That it was not a serendipity occurrence for Miss. Minnie T. Gore, the Director of Homer G. Phillips Nursing School, provided me with the opportunity to return to nursing school after we were married. I believe it was spiritually motivated. Baby, I know along my journey of becoming a nurse, the right people were placed in my life's path at the right time, which allowed me to fulfill my spiritual calling to become a nurse.

Willis, I have had a wonderful, satisfying, and successful nursing career overall. I was a dedicated and effective nurse, and I fulfilled my dream of being a "good" nurse; I provided nursing services as an operating room nurse, St. Louis Visiting Public Health Nurse; servicing young expecting mothers that were frightened from uncertainty about their future moving forward with their lives.

I was a psych nurse working in a private-sector hospital in St. Louis. Also, I was particularly a caring psychiatric nurse in the VA hospital system. I was able to assist military veterans in overcoming their emotional and mental situations and, most of all, the VA women struggling with their sexual abuse in the military.

From a cogent point of view, regardless of how insignificant some may deem it to have been. Through my successes, I persevered through trials and tribulations with self-confidence and the love of my family. I didn't accomplish becoming the nurse that I am of my own volition. Remarkably, the help and sacrifices that Momma and mother Drake provided me with were invaluable. I remember Mother Drake's statement when I was pregnant with Monica, that I would be a wonderful nurse. Willis, I believe I have lived up to mother Drake's proclamation that day!

Willis, I know that plans for my life were directed; otherwise, I wouldn't have been blessed as abundantly as I am." Smiling broadly, I acknowledged her sentiments without saying a word, that Mary was blessed and "Destined and Determined" to be a nurse.

MDI (Male Duck Incorporated) Bound:
As we were finishing eating dinner, I told Mary jokingly, I know you will assume your official role as the MDI office manager. Now I don't want you coming in trying to do things differently. Laughing, she said, man, I am going to set up my own filing system that I am familiar with,

so I don't want to hear anything about it. We laughed as Mary cleaned up the kitchen.

Mary came from a highly active nursing career that was mentally stimulating and professionally satisfying. She needed, metaphorically speaking, a cooling down period from her nursing job. She was not prepared to relegate herself to idle time and unproductive activity, so the bridge from her VA position to the MDI office manager job was on point.

I retired in 2001 and was operating MDI with my son Kermit. The land-scape had been laid for the last six months before Mary retired; for her to immediately take over the role and responsibilities as secretary-treasurer and office manager for MDI. Following her retirement, Mary was expecting to integrate into MDI's management to assist with operating our small (business) multi-million dollar company.

I established MDI in 1988 as a family-owned small business. First, MDI started with my father's inspiration when I was 15 years old, and he suggested that my brothers and I start a family business. From that time, I visualized my ideas, drafted them on paper, and put them into a plan that became a reality.

Sometimes an idea, vision, or dream can only be imagined by the be-holder. The first product I created was "making buttons" with slogans I had created (written), trademarked, and copyrighted. I then purchased a single-button press-machine maker that I had seen advertised on tele-vision. I then had an artist friend, John Joiner, with whom I had attend-ed Eugene Field Elementary School and Charles Sumner High School while living in St. Louis, Missouri. John drew the written slogans and designs I had created to a physical scale object.

I recall vividly working on the dining room table as my workbench when we lived at 7204 Neaptide Lane in Burke, Virginia. With no experience or knowledge, by trial and error, I used the single button press-machine maker to press out "3-inch buttons," which had my design slogans print-ed on them.

As I established MDI as a bootstrap company operation, my first Enterprise was making "Buttons and T-Shirts Designs." I peddled my wearers (products) to street vendors in Washington, DC. Mostly a vendor named Joe Shelton had a vendor stand at 12th and F streets on the weekends. He always had a vendor stand in front of the Washington DC District Building at the Fourth Street intersection during the week.

My T-shirts and the 12th man Buttons had my logo of MDI on them. A Male Duck is a "Drake" my surname is Drake. Therefore, I incorporated my business as "Male Duck Incorporated." Joe would always call me "Duck," and when he met Mary, he called her Mrs. Duck.

Following that T-shirts and Buttons enterprise, I created a multi-million dollar consulting firm supporting federal government projects and contracts. This was my vision since my father planted the seed in my mind when I was 15 years old. Over the years, Mary shared in my vision, as I shared in her dream and goal to be a nurse.

Now MDI is operated mainly by its president, Kermit Matthew Drake, the Executive Vice President, Willis Drake, and its Secretary-Treasurer and office manager, Mary Ann Byas-Drake.

My daughter Monica Drake-Zinn and my son-in-law Gordon Zinn had worked for MDI also.

Mary handled the company's payroll, federal, state, and local taxes, insurance, and normal HR (Human Resource) day-to-day office-related operations. Her functions were a "Vital and significant viable part of our small business."

The executive vice president managed the day-to-day technical and policy issues. MDI is an 8a-certified company with a GSA Mission Oriented Business Integrated Services (MOBIS) Contract in force for twenty years.

Initially, I handled the preparation of our "C corporate taxes (Form 1120)" when we were only producing and selling T-shirts and Buttons. However, during the peak years of operating MDI at various periods, we employed sixteen personnel in eight states (Virginia, Ohio, New York, Chicago, Georgia, Pennsylvania, Florida, and New Jersey).

Therefore MDI had to hire the services of a Certified Public Accountant (CPA) to file our corporate income tax for the federal, state, and local governments. We were fortunate to be introduced to Ms. Marva Benn, a CPA. She lived in our general area in Fairfax Station, Virginia. She came with a high reference from a friend, Tessa Murphy, who was a coworker at mobile oil with Marva.

Marva Benn, MDI's CPA
Initially, Marva and I worked together on the taxes. At the time, MDI's income was so small that preparing our taxes was not complex, and Marva's tax services, cost-wise, were basically complementary. Our conversations concerning the taxes were brief. Then MDI was awarded multiple government contracts that propelled MDI's annual income into the multimillion-dollar income range.

Mary and Marva, professionally and personally, immediately hit it off very well, working together. Now, our tax withholding process has expanded due to the increased income. Instead of reporting our taxes quarterly, we now had to report our tax withholdings bi-weekly. As office manager, Mary had to coordinate with the IRS (Internal Revenue Service) and put in place a bi-weekly income tax withholding process for Social Security and federal, state, and local income tax for our employees.

Mary ordered a payroll and tax software system (QuickBooks) that she used and coordinated with Marva so that the yearend assesses and corporate taxes would be in sync. Mary and Marva would be on the phone for hours talking. The phone call was supposedly initiated to make a quick reference for information concerning MDI that only would require a few minutes to obtain or verify. However, literally, an hour later, Mary and Marva would still be on the phone talking, laughing, and having an interesting conversation.

So our business relationship with Marva evolved into more of a personal and family relationship. We got to know one another's families. We

met Marva's mother and father; attended her daughter, Akiva Olure-
mi Kirkland's (Remi Kirkland) wedding; got to follow her grandson,
Joseph Donovan Beal's (Jo-Jo) school development as he went off to
college, and the birth of her granddaughter, Sydney Corinne Kirkland.

Mary would convey to me how Marva would raise MDI, as this small
company had negative income taxes to report when she started working
with us. Then, within a couple of years, we were reporting an annual
gross income of 4 million dollars, and she would exclaim how I had
built the business from this T-shirt and Button operation. She knew how
blessed we were with our government consulting contractor support
business operations being so successful.

I was more business-minded, and when Marva came to the house to
have me sign our corporate tax form (Form 1120), it would take five
minutes, but then Mary and Marva would socialize for hours. I could
always depend on Marva to prepare our taxes, but sometimes she would
be close to the deadline date, and she and Mary just seemed cavalier
about it, whereas I was more anxious.

MDI created a reputation for completing its assignments on time and
fulfilling its contracts within scope and costs. Mary Ann Byas-Drake
was a large part of MDI's operation, and Marva Benn, as our CPA, con-
tributed to MDI's success. More than her professional services, Marva's
personal friendship has been invaluable.

I had anticipated the time when Mary and I would be retired. We were
active and productive in our part-time jobs with MDI. We gradual-
ly engaged in doing fun things we enjoyed and still work for MDI.
We were blessed to take one week out of each ten or eleven months
during the year and travel to a favorite location we enjoyed visiting
and spending time.

Mary's journey with MDI's development was commensurate with her
effort to become a registered nurse. She and I were both blessed to see
the dreams we each had fostered during our lifetime come to fruition
and be fulfilled.

CHAPTER 39

———— ◇ ————

Mary's Appreciation Celebration Dinner

———— ◇ ————

IN AUGUST 2009, MARY ANN Byas-Drake and I were within eight months of being married for fifty years. Therefore, unequivocally based on longevity alone, I could confirm that she is truly a kind-hearted and caring person. Consequently, that was why Mary's family (brothers, sisters, aunts, cousins, nieces, and nephews) honored her for what she had done for them during their lifetime.

Mary's family now had this phenomenal opportunity to show their appreciation for her impact on each of their lives. Often time's, opportunities like this escape us. That happens when we put off acknowledging a person in this fashion while they are still among the living.

In the East St. Louis area, at least generationally, Mary's family acknowledged her as the current family's matriarch. She was the oldest female cousin, and the young cousins, in concert with Mary's nieces, had aspirations to emulate her. Throughout her lifetime, Mary was a revered daughter, mother, sister, niece, aunt, cousin, and a good friend to many she had encountered.

Mary was indeed a "big sister," being nine years older than her two younger brothers and two young sisters. She was like a teenage mother figure looking out for her siblings growing up. She would cuddle and praise her two young sisters when they were preschoolers, and she was a positive influence as they became teenagers.

Moreover, she was "down to earth" and loved being around her family. She related positively with her young brothers as well. Personally, she had fun as a teenager, and she enjoyed music, listening, and singing, as well as dancing, and she would quickly learn the latest dance steps. She demonstrated her lady qualities doing it!

As an adult, she could engage in hyperbole girl-talk conversations, yet she could hold an intellectual discussion on local and national political issues and world events. Yet, she was still comfortable engaging in the gossip headlines of the local or expose newspapers. Her family members from all perspectives of life confided in her and could relate to her very comfortably. She did not criticize or judge anyone or embarrass them publicly.

She didn't seek recognition for any notable charitable deeds that she rendered. Rather, she would anonymously accomplish her benevolence or bless her family members privately, with no fanfare, acknowledgment, or expected return benefits. What she did was from the goodness of her heart.

Just maybe it was Mary's genuine temperament that allowed her to extend her generosity to others in ways that positively affected their lives. Possibly, her profession as a registered nurse spilled over into her everyday life requiring her to care for her family and friends in a distinct way. Regardless, her desire to help others was not a burden or impediment for her. Rather, her professional contemporaries and personal friends always commended her for helping others the way that she did.

The Guest Arrives!
The temperature was sweltering that August morning in Triangle, Virginia, compared to how the month of July had ended temperature-wise. Preparing to travel, Mary was scurrying about upstairs, then downstairs, to get herself ready. Traditionally, she would pack her suitcase well in advance of her travel departure date.

However, preparing to travel for this trip, Mary's frantic actions started to fray my nerves, and finally, I said, "baby, just relax. However, my words landed on deaf ears. She pretended not to be nervous and, with a fictitious smile on her face, told me humorously to mind my own business. "Willis, I will be packed and ready to go before you are packed, so please don't bother me."

Now I just observed Mary silently as she was getting packed to travel to her hometown, "East St. Louis, Illinois." In a few days, she would be back in her old stomping grounds to be the guest of honor at her "Appreciation Celebration Dinner." The hostesses primarily were her sisters Mona (Wooten) and Margaret Ann (Franklin).

I knew how important the affair was for Mary. I also understood her nervousness, knowing in precisely three days, this event would take place. Within her overall family structure, she was now the cornerstone of her generation. She represented the moral fabric and inspiration and provided an example for the young family members to model their lives.

As the night drew near, I finished packing my suitcase. Mary was checking for last-minute items she wanted to take with her. In a soft tone, "Baby, you don't have enough space in your suitcase to take all your clothes, okay."

Without saying a word, Mary's movements became defter, as she finished packing and zipped up her suitcase. Looking at me with a little agitation, she said" Willis, you can take my suitcase downstairs now." Trying to ease the aggravation I had caused, I responded, okay, sweetheart, and posthaste I carried our luggage downstairs.

I was somewhat hyper, too, thinking of journeying to St. Louis, where our entire families would be attending Mary's Appreciation Celebration Dinner on Saturday, August 8th. However, beforehand, and without focus, I would celebrate my sixty-ninth birthday on Friday, August 7th.

When I returned to the bedroom, I could hear Mary getting ready for bed in the bathroom. I tried to lighten the tension in the air that I had caused. When she entered the bedroom, I went and hugged and kissed her. Those active gestures seemed to break the "ice" positively, and now Mary was smiling. She said, "Don't try to get friendly now after rushing me to pack my suitcase." However, she was not resisting my embrace, and I sincerely apologized if I had upset her.

We both were now stirring around, getting ready for bed. It was still early, and I certainly was not ready to go to sleep. In a suggestive tone, I asked, "Mary are you coming to bed soon?" I could hear her snickering in a light-hearted way. It was a casual reflective response as she said, "what's on your mind, man? Are you expecting an early birthday present?"

She had a broad smile that suddenly became an outburst of happy laughter. Babe, after all these years, you still think you have that magic touch; come on, admit it. She continued to laugh, saying your loving affection would overwhelm me then, and I must admit, yes, old man, you still have that persuasive presence about you. I was silent, but the smile on my face said it all. Laying in bed, my ego was multiplied a thousand times.

She was now standing on her side of the bed; I stretched out my hand, inviting her to bed. Excitingly, she grasped and tightly held my hand as she slid under the bed covers, and we embraced. Following a blissful night, I woke up in the morning, and Mary's back was towards me, and I nudged closer to her and whispered in her ear. My soft voice was more for effect than for privacy, as we were alone in the house. I gently touched her face, rubbing her soft cheeks as I often did. I then said softly, wake up, sleepyhead.

Enticing Mary to wake up was effective. Slowly she turned over, facing me as her smile caressed her face. Yawning with her arms stretched out, she said, "I know it's not time to get up already." She reached and put her left arm around my neck, pulling me closer to her. I smiled and said, "sleepy head; we have a plane to catch this morning; you need to hurry and get up."

Now she was out of bed and staring off into space. It was a gaze that I had not seen before. Then she turned quickly, looking at me, and instantly I could see the moisture in her eyes. She said, "Willis, I am so blessed to have my family honoring me with this appreciation dinner on Saturday.

Babe, for me, emotionally, it is overwhelming just thinking of my little sisters, and yes, my brothers David and Terry, too, spearheading this event and gathering the support of my entire family. It is a tremendous expression of their love for me." Mary was obviously excited, anticipating her special event.

Wiping her eyes with her right hand, she quickly moved from the bedside. Talking to herself, she said, "okay, I need to get moving. I don't want to be late for our flight to St. Louis." Then talking aloud, Willis, I got a reservation at the Marriott Airport Hotel, where we like to stay.

Checking the clock, "Hey, we are getting pressed for time. Do you want to shower first, or should I get mine now?" Mary looked at me without responding as if I had untowardly dismissed her comment about the hotel reservation. She quickly moved toward the bathroom to take her shower.

To take advantage of time, while Mary was taking her shower, I was shaving and brushing my teeth in the outer bathroom area. Looking in the mirror, I was reminiscing when Mary's sister, Romona (Mona), first called to tell me of the plans to give "Pookie" an "Appreciation Dinner."

Mona explained with excitement that all of "Pookie's" siblings and their entire family (aunt, cousins, nieces, and nephews) wanted to honor Pookie for all she had done, throughout her life, for their entire family. Mona wanted to confirm a date that would be available for Pookie and me and for our children and grandchildren to attend the Appreciation Dinner.

As I finished shaving, I had a smile on my face, and I snapped back to the present time. I called out to Mary, who was still in the shower, "Okay baby, I know you enjoy taking long relaxing showers, but let's hurry up, please. We have a plane to catch this morning."

Then I heard Mary's familiar retort with attitude in her voice. "Man, don't rush me, I will be done when I am done, and you get on my nerves." It sounded like her voice was reverberating above the splashing water from the shower. Hearing Mary's voice, I concealed my laughter, and I could hardly wait until she got out of the shower.

I heard the water stop running in the shower, and Mary said, "Willis are you finished out there now? You have been rushing me, and I need my privacy. So will you get out of here so I can get dressed?" I laughed and said, "Just hurry up." Then her familiar response rang out, "man, don't be rushing me." I was laughing under my breath as I left the bathroom.

It didn't take Mary long to finish in the bathroom. Shortly, she entered the bedroom, and I immediately went and got my shower. We both were hurriedly getting dressed, as there was a sense of urgency in getting to the airport on time.

Routinely we used the BWI (Baltimore Washington International) Airport in Baltimore, Maryland. In normal traffic, it would take us approximately one and a half hours to drive to BWI. We also calculated the time to park our car in the airport parking garage and catch the shuttle bus to Southwest Airlines' terminal to be on time for our flight.

When possible, we traveled on Southwest Airlines and always had pre-boarding (priority) seating arrangements. We would sit on the left side of the airplane in rows nine, ten, or eleven. Mary preferred the window seat, and I would sit in the aisle seat. When the airplane was not completely full, and the middle seat was vacant between us, we would have a really comfortable flight.

This morning we had arrived in plenty of time at the airport, and Mary was able to purchase breakfast at the terminal to take on the plane. We were among the first passengers to board the airplane that morning, and we settled comfortably before the plane took off.

There were few passengers on this flight, as the airplane was only half full. Mary had adequate space in the overhead storage compartment to put her dress bag, containing the dress she would wear Saturday evening to her affair. Mary had the dress made by a local seamstress in Springfield, Virginia. She did not want to wrinkle her dress in the airplane's overhead baggage storage compartment.

As the airplane was taking off, Mary and I confirmed the flight time from BWI to St. Louis was one hour and 55 minutes. Routinely, I would be asleep, sometimes before the airplane would lift off from the runway. Mary normally would have headphones on, listening to music.

However, this flight was different for me. I was wide awake when the airplane roared down the runway, and the wheels lifted off the ground. Mary held my hand and said, "how beautiful the sky was as the plane ascended effortlessly toward its flight altitude." Then we heard the flight attendant announce that "you could move about the cabinet but while seated to keep your seatbelt fastened."

Gazing at me, she said, "Babe, I am surprised you are not asleep already." Smiling, I acknowledged my surprise also that I was still awake. I reached over and touched her face, saying, "I was excited and just couldn't sleep before the airplane got airborne this morning."

Spontaneously, I kissed Mary lightly and said "girl I love you." Mary smiling like the teenager she was in my mind's eye view, said softly, "I am so thankful for you and the family that we have. For them to orchestrate this wonderful event for me is overwhelmingly wonderful. Willis, we have a loving family."

At that moment, I agreed wholeheartedly with Mary, and I didn't have to say a word. Then my thoughts advanced to my imagination, knowing that, literally, Mary would be able to smell the roses, metaphorically speaking, in real time. Also, she would actually "hear the kind words of thanks and appreciation that would be articulated about her during her "Appreciation Dinner." While she is still alive, to have her family honoring her in this distinct wonderful way was gracious by her family.

Our plane would touch down in St. Louis in an hour. So I reclined my seat back and closed my eyes to catch a nap during the remainder of the flight. When the plane landed, we got our luggage from the overhead compartment. Mary was clutching her dress bag as I got the suitcases. With our luggage in hand, we boarded the shuttle bus to pick up our rental car.

With our Budget "Fastbreak" reservation, we quickly picked up the rental car and drove to the Marriott St. Louis Airport Hotel. The rental agency was only five minutes away, and we arrived at the hotel and had an early check-in. Shortly after we entered the room, we immediately crashed to take a nap.

For this trip, we arrived in town on Thursday morning; so we would have time to visit with family and friends during our short stay in town. Several hours later that afternoon, we woke up and went and visited my brother Melvin Drake and his wife, Shirley. We had not seen them this year, so we talked excessively for several hours, just catching up on everything. Shirley said that their family (she, Melvin, Dana, and Delaney) would be at the affair.

Melvin and I had our conversation as Shirley and Mary were catching up on everything. It was customary when we visited my brother's house to break bread as Shirley had prepared a light lunch. We enjoyed the food and conversation visiting with my big brother and sister-in-law.

Leaving Melvin's house, I programmed my GPS (Global Positioning System) for directions to the Lake Charles Park Cemetery. Whenever I visit St. Louis, I always visit my parent's and my aunt Tee's (Ethel Mae Sanford's) gravesites.

We left the cemetery and stopped at my sister Joan Harris' home. Seeing Joan and her husband Bobby (Flarzell Harris) was always a stop we made when in St. Louis. We had planned only a brief visit. However, we were talking, laughing, and enjoying ourselves; as a result, we were at their home much longer than planned. Now we were rushing again, and we had to travel to East St. Louis during the downtown St. Louis rush-hour traffic.

Mary was clear that she wanted to stop first, for a minute, at Aunt Alleen's (Byas) house when we got to East St. Louis. It was approaching 4:30 pm when we arrived at her home. When Aunt Alleen opened the door, she immediately gave Mary a tremendous hug. It was very obvious how glad she was to see both of us.

We returned Aunt Alleen's warm greetings, and Mary told her we just wanted to put our feet inside her home; however, we would only stay a few minutes. Mary reminded her aunt, "I will see you on Saturday evening, and we can talk and catch up then."

We left Aunt Alleen's house and went directly to Mary's brother David's house. When we pulled up in front of David's house, he came out immediately and opened the car door for his big sister, Pookie.

David was towering over his big sister outside the car as they hugged and greeted one another. Looking at the two of them embrace, I could tell that Mary's big sister's demeanor was still apparent to younger brother David!

David and I greeted one another; as we shook hands, he said, "Hey Will" let's go inside; it's still hot out here. We retreated to the house; Mary and David were catching up on how his kids, A'Ryanne and Dierdre (Dee Dee), and their families were doing.

David said in his normal dry humor, "What do you mean, kids; my grandkids will soon be adults." He was now laughing as he dialogued with his sister, "Pookie."

Mary, laughing, also said, "I am feeling like an old lady when I see our next generation of young folks." With his trademark toothpick in his mouth, David said, "you will see them at the dinner Saturday evening." Then in a serious tone of voice, David said, "Pookie, you and Will have done so much for all of us. You deserve every bit of our thanks and appreciation."

With some emotion on her face, Mary said, all shucks David, "We were just doing what we could." Standing up, she said well, we had better hit the road, so we can stop to see Margaret Ann for a few minutes. Then, we will stick our heads in to see Mona and Steve on our way back to St. Louis. You know, unless I had arranged with your brother Terry in advance, it would be hard to catch up with him. I will be out of luck seeing him this evening.

We left David's house to go to Margaret Ann's home. Mary talked with her earlier on the phone, and she was expecting us. I was sitting in the living room chair as big sister and little sister engaged in conversation and laughter. Margaret Ann told Mary that her son Jason (Franklin) was doing well. They hugged, and we said goodbye. Mary said, "We will see you and Jason on Saturday."

We were now on our way to Mona and her husband Steve's (Rev. Steve Wooten) home. She wanted to make sure that Mona didn't need her help with anything for Saturday evening's affair. When we arrived at the house, Stephanie, Mary's niece, opened the door. She said hi Aunt Pookie and Uncle Willis in her soft voice as she hugged her aunt. She obviously was excited seeing her aunt, Pookie.

Mona hearing her big sister Pookie's unique patterned laugh, she came into the living room and hugged her. Steve was sitting on the couch watching television. After we had greeted one another, Mary and Mona retreated to the dining room to have their personal conversation. Steve and I sat on the couch watching TV and chitchatted a bit.

Ten minutes later, Mary and Mona came into the living room, and Mary was laughing as she said, "Willis, everything is under control," and she and Mona hugged again. Steve and I also had to laugh as well. Seeing little sister Mona affirming to her big sister Pookie, "I got this," you can just relax. Steve and I appreciated the moment as we slapped hands.

Mary and I left their house at 7:00 pm. The long day was starting to set in on us, and we were ready to return to the hotel. However, first, we had to make our normal stop at our favorite Chinese restaurant for our Chinese food take-out, for dinner back to the hotel.

The restaurant owner would always say to Mary, "You are from Virginia." She and Mary would exchange pleasantries, and our Chinese food order was always packed overly full. The restaurant was ten minutes from the Marriott hotel.

Now back in our hotel room, we got comfortable and started eating dinner. I would eat my entire Chinese meal. Mary would talk while eating, and she liked her food hot. So she would reheat her food in the microwave before she finished eating. She usually would only eat half of her food and put the rest in the refrigerator to eat later.

It was a few minutes past 10 o'clock when we finished dinner and went to bed. I don't remember anything after my head hit the pillow. I was "comping zees" as I fell into slumberland immediately.

I woke up at 7:30 am the following day, which was late for me. Mary was still asleep, and it was an hour and a half later before she woke up. Sitting up in bed, displaying her patent smile and a good morning pierced her lips. She asked how long have you been up, babe? Did you sleep well last night? Responding, with a smile on my face, "Hey, I slept very well like I was in my bed at home."

I was sitting in the chair at the desk next to the TV. Mary pivoted to the side of the bed and got up. She was now standing as she stretched and yawned, with her arms extended towards the ceiling. She walked towards the bathroom, and as she passed by me, she rubbed my face softly. When she came out of the bathroom, she still had not said "happy birthday" to me.

My Birthday
Instead, she started a casual conversation asking me, "what was the temperature like outside this morning?" This trivial conversation may have been due to thinking about her event tomorrow night instead of remembering today is my birthday. Sitting at the desk, I was waiting for those two simple words "Happy Birthday" to ring in my ears.

Now thirty minutes had elapsed since Mary was awake and up. She still had not wished me a happy birthday! My patience had waned, and in an upset voice, I said, "You do know today is my birthday, and you have not wished me happy birthday yet!"

Smiling and recognizing her oversight, she was immediately apologetic. Mary came over, sat on my lap, put her arms around my neck, and said sincerely, "I am so sorry, babe. Happy birthday, Happy birthday! I promise that I will make it up to you." Her eyes were bright, and she said don't forget your "rain check" for your birthday. She kissed me, and we were all good as we went about getting our day started.

It was a fortuitous situation; my birthday was this weekend. However, there was no added emphasis placed on celebrating my birthday. However, if we did not have dinner, we as a family would follow our family tradition, have cake, and ice cream to celebrate my birthday.

Now wide awake, Mary and I went through our normal routine, asking who would take a shower first. However, we ended up just lounging in the hotel room until past noon time. Mary watched her favorite TV programs, and we made phone calls to friends and family members, letting them know we were in town. Subsequently, Mary got her shower first, and then I got mine.

Willis Jr., Monica, and Kermit Matthew and their families would arrive in St. Louis later that evening. Our children were staying at a different hotel, only 10 minutes away from the Marriott Hotel where we were staying. Our daughter Monica called and let us know that everyone had arrived in town and registered at their hotel.

Our kids were planning to take us to dinner for my birthday and asked if we would be ready in have dinner in an hour. Now Mary was rushing to get ready, so she could see the kids. We left our hotel, and minutes later, we were at the hotel where the children were staying.

We entered the hotel, and the kids were waiting in the lobby for us. Our granddaughter, Adriana, rushed to meet her grandmother. It was good to see Adriana, Monica, and her husband Gordon, who lives in Sagamore Hills, Ohio, near Cleveland. We saw Willis Jr. and his wife Marilyn more often; they lived in Brunswick, MD, an hour and a half from us. Kermit, his wife Danita, and their eleven-month-old daughter Déjà resided in Woodbridge, VA, ten minutes from us.

After the hugs and hellos, Mary extracted Déjà from Danita's arms to hold her. Now, attention was directed at wishing me a "happy birthday." We laughed about me "getting old." Then quickly, the focus switched as everybody was excited about the Appreciation Dinner tomorrow for their mother.

Now it was getting near dinner time, and Mary holding Déjà in her arms, said, okay, I am hungry; let's go to a restaurant close by the hotel for dinner. During dinner, we laughed, reminisced fondly about past times, and had a terrific, gaiety, low-key dinner. After dinner, Mary had Monica buy a birthday cake and ice cream, and we returned to the kid's hotel to celebrate my birthday.

We gathered in the hotel room where Monica's family was staying. In our family birthday tradition, the family "Sang happy birthday; I made my wish, and blew out my birthday candles." The luck came if you blew out all the candles in one breath. For this birthday, I had 70 candles to blow out, sixty-nine for my age, and one to grow on.

Following this tradition, I cut the first (large) slice of cake and had a big scoop of ice cream. Mary then cut the cake for everyone, and Adriana put a scoop of ice cream on their plates. We talked, joked, and ate our cake and ice cream. Then as the evening wound down, I read my birthday cards privately I received from Mary, family members, and friends.

As twilight approached, semidarkness appeared on the horizon. Mary said to me, "babe, you look tired, are you ready to go back to the hotel?" I immediately understood her non-verbal cue and responded, "yes, it's 9:00 o'clock already, and we should go back to our hotel." I gathered my birthday cards and thanked the kids for a wonderful 69th birthday celebration.

We left the hotel and returned to our Marriott hotel rather quickly, settling in for the night. Mary and I were laughing and talking as we were getting ready for bed. She said, "babe, I hope you enjoyed your birthday celebration. I know the kids, and I did." Before responding, I reflected deeply on the personal words written on my birthday cards from Mary and the kids.

Then I assured her, "yes, sweetheart, I really had a wonderful 69th birthday. Our family being together was the best birthday gift I could have received. Also, that store-bought birthday cake tasted really good too. You know how I like my sweets." Smiling, Mary said, "yes, you know I always take care of you. I brought you a big slice of cake to eat later."

Now lying in bed on my 69th birthday, Mary had her head resting on my chest. That was a familiar place where she felt most comfortable, and it represented closeness between us that had matured over the forty-nine years we were married.

Mary raised her head from my chest. Looking at me, she gently pulled my head down and whispered in my ear, "happy birthday, Willis." She smiled as she said, "you know I don't renege on my promises! Are you up to receive your birthday present now?" I was laughing confidently, and I responded softly, "absolutely" you know I never refuse your birthday present anytime! Our night ended blissfully.

Anticipating the August 8, 2009 Event
I woke up feeling great, and I slid out of bed quietly. I was cautious not to disturb Mary as she was still sound asleep. I decided to postpone taking my shower and getting dressed until Mary awakens. Gazing down at her sleeping, I relished in the comfort of our togetherness. I also reminisced about last night, and the wonderful evening I had with my children and their families, celebrating my 69th birthday. I felt so blessed as the family patriarch.

I sat in the chair at the desk and meditated reflectively. I was observing Mary in slumberland resting so peacefully. The weight of getting ready to participate in her event over the past few days had evaporated from her countenance. She was asleep with a pleasant smile on her face.

Mary's life's actions these past many years would culminate tonight with her family's glorious recognition of love for their "Pookie."

My eyes were still on Mary lying in bed. It was now a little past noon, and I wanted her to sleep as long as possible before I woke her up. I had to jolt myself mentally to finally wake her up. I knew this evening would be enjoyable for her, but I also knew it would be a long, emotional, and exhausting evening also.

I gently tickled her face, creating a slight annoyance to awaken her. Instinctively, Mary swatted softly at her face, and a frown appeared as she started to awaken. She opened her eyes and, still half asleep, asked what time it was. Touching my hand, and stating clearly, Willis, you know I can sleep a lot longer. Responding softly, sleepyhead, it is already noon; yes, I know you can sleep all day without any problem.

Mary sat up in the bed and casually said, "Good morning, babe; how did you sleep?" Laughing, "Girl, I slept fine, and I was able to get up early this morning as usual too. It seems that you need time to recover to get up this morning." We both laughed and admitted that responding the next morning at age 68 or 69 is different from when we were eighteen and nineteen.

I told Mary, "if you are hungry, I will treat you to lunch. Therefore you will need to get a shower and get dressed to go out to eat." Getting out of bed, Mary said Willis, I think I will order a tossed salad and a cheeseburger from the hotel's restaurant. I like their food, and they will put lots of onions on my cheeseburger the way I like it. Will you go get my food and bring it back to the room for me?

Babe, I plan to just lounge around in my pajamas until it is time to get dressed for tonight. Having a salad and a cheeseburger for lunch will hold me until around 7:00 o'clock tonight, when dinner probably will be served.

I went down to the hotel restaurant, and there were only a few people; I ordered a tossed salad and cheeseburger. The waitress asked, "Do you want French fries too?" "No thanks." The waitress returned in 15 minutes with my order, and I was back in our room in 20 minutes.

Mary was sitting in the middle of the bed watching TV when I got back to the room. I gave her the bag with her food. She said, "This cheeseburger smells really good." Then she took the Toss Salad from the bag and said, "Willis, this is a huge salad; can you please eat half of it?"

I had gotten hungry smelling Mary's food, and I took half of the salad and sat in the chair at the desk, and we ate lunch. We watched television and relaxed and talked to pass time. When I checked the time, to my surprise, it was 4:00 o'clock.

Having finished eating, Mary was sitting in the middle of the bed. She was relaxing with two pillows propping her up, and she looked very comfortable. With a sense of alarm, "what time do you want to leave this evening?" Remember, it may take you a little longer to get dressed tonight for the affair.

Mary sprung out of bed, walked over, and opened her suitcase. With a coy smile on her face, she said, "Willis, don't worry, I will be ready in plenty of time." Mary's proactive approach at this moment caught me off guard. I asked her if she wanted me to take my shower first. She responded quickly, "yes, babe, go ahead and get your shower. I will get my clothes laid out and organized while you are taking your shower."

Earlier that morning, I decided I would be "cool" and not aggravate Mary while she was getting ready. However, she did not need any prompting from me. She inspected every piece of garment she laid out to wear. I teased her about looking "fly" in her tailored made dress. We were both dressed in sufficient time and just relaxed before leaving the hotel.

I suggested leaving a few minutes early in case something unexpected was to happen on the way to the golf course. Confidently Mary said, "Willis, I have a general idea where the golf course is located. When I was in high school, I recall prominent professional and affluent African-Americans living in East St. Louis talking about Grand Maria's Golf Course.

Research shows it was built in 1938 and was one of eight **Black-owned golf courses in the United States.** It was probably one of the nicer places in East St. Louis during that time. The East St. Louis African-American community patronized the golf course well. I remember it is located on Lake Drive; we should not have any problem finding it.

As we left the hotel room, Mary was holding my right arm while walking to the elevator. This was normally what she did when we were together. Now getting off the elevator and walking through the hotel lobby, I feel proud with Mary clutching my arm and looking good.

It was a short walk to the car, and Mary particularly did not want to get her dressed wrinkled unnecessarily, getting in the car. Now comfortable in the car, she said, "Willis, please turn on the air conditioner. I don't want to start perspiring in this heat."

Mary was silent for a minute, staring straight ahead with an uncertain look on her face. I could not discern if her expression was from having doubt about her event tonight. "The Grand Maria's Lighthouse Restaurant was located at **5802 Lake Dr, East Saint Louis.** I plugged the address into my GPS.

Leaving the hotel, the temperature was close to 90 degrees. The air conditioner was kicking on high as we entered highway I-70 East. I was teasing Mary a little bit, saying, "girl your dinner affair is being held at a prestigious location in East St. Louis. When you grace the premises this evening, I am sure the establishment will be upgraded more. We laughed as we drove to Grand Maria's Golf Course without difficulty.

Mary was still somewhat overcome by this appreciation dinner in her honor. She extolled the fact that so many family members would be attending the affair. Smiling, she said, "Mona told me that Juanita Rupert-Russell and Phyllis McNeese-McReynolds, my two best childhood friends will also be attending tonight. Willis, the thought of their presence on this occasion warms my heart.

We arrived half an hour early and waited in the car to stay cool. Mary was calm, cool, and collected as we waited 15 minutes in the parking lot. I drove Mary to the restaurant's front entrance, so she could avoid walking in the heat. Getting out of the car, she said, "thanks, babe; I will wait in the restaurant lobby for you."

I parked the car and hurried to the restaurant to avoid the heat myself. It was now fifteen minutes before the affair was to start. Mary was waiting in the restaurant's foyer. When I reached her, she encompassed my right arm, as we walked into the restaurant.

Immediately, as we entered the restaurant, our granddaughter Adriana and four great-nieces, Amber, Stephanie, Cecily, and Arin, called out in unison, "Aunt Pookie," as they advanced toward us, practically running. I disengaged Mary from my arm to allow Aunt Pookie's girls to greet her. Mary was a little cautious in the hugs and embraces, not wanting to get her dress wrinkled.

The girls were talking at once, wanting to get their Aunt Pookie's attention. Finally surrounding her and holding her hands, they led Aunt Pookie to a table where she could sit. I joined Mary there and got the customary hi, Uncle Willis. These were Aunt Pookie's girls, and her other two girls, Terrianna and Keyarra had not arrived yet.

Quickly, Aunt Pookie's girls returned to putting tablecloths and the gift centerpiece arrangements on the tables. Now, as the guests started to arrive, seeing Mary, they were immediately drawn to the table where Mary was sitting.

It was heartwarming for me to see the admiration and genuine love expressed toward Mary. The restaurant was filling up, and family members that spanned four generations of Mary's family showed up. Mary's friends were there, and three generations of my family were also present to honor their "Aunt Mary."

The affair would start in a few minutes, and Mary's sisters Mona and Margaret Ann escorted Mary, me, our children, and their families to the head table as honored guests.

As the evening unfolded, the occasion was wonderful. Mary's cousin Paulette Tolden was the mistress of ceremony. Mary's siblings each gave a verbal tribute to their big sister, as well as other family members and friends did also. The food was delicious, and the atmosphere was fantastic.

However, for me, the highlight of the evening was the tribute in songs performed by Mary's cousin Jo Jo (Ardella Lovelace-Miller), who sang: His Eye Is On The Sparrow, and Three Times A Lady. Mary's childhood friend Phyllis McNeese-McReynolds sang the song: Precious Lord Take My Hand. Phyllis' performance inspired the guests to join in singing along with her, and that was a very spiritual time of the celebration.

Then the preverbal icing on the cake was Mary's "Thank you remarks" to her family and friends. She was humorous and articulate, with a sense of humility and genuineness in her comments. Her overarching appreciation stating that "each of you would take your time to come out and participate in this affair honoring me in this way, shows the love you have for me. I greatly appreciate each of you."

Those verbal sentiments and the personal thank you from Mary to each person who attended the affair capped off the wonderful occasion for her. She basically hugged and kissed all her guests. As we were leaving the restaurant, that was a day to remember for the rest of our lives. It was not surprising to me because Mary was "Destined and Determined" for many things in her life. After having an exceptional enjoyable affair in Mary's honor; we all returned home safely!

CHAPTER 40

Mary's Peritoneal Dialysis Treatment

W HEN MARY RETIRED FROM THE VA, she settled into a comfortable retirement routine as she slide into her role at MDI as a part-time employee. The demands of MDI for Mary's time and my time were equivalent to having a small part-time job. We both worked when we needed to conduct essential MDI company business for our retirement lives going forward.

At this point in our lives, Mary and I enjoyed spending time with one another and our collective family members. Our basic retirement scenario included us traveling to areas in the United States, the Caribbean islands, and specific places where our family members resided. We were blessed with the opportunity to enjoy life in a modest way that was personally satisfying for us.

We were enjoying our retirement life, taking in local stage plays and music concerts, going to art museums, attending Broadway plays in New York City, and traveling to exciting locations with our close friends, Charles and Emma Smith. We started shortly after Mary retired in 2004, embarked upon traveling, and engaged in the things we enjoyed doing together.

Entering into our retirement, I provided the MDI corporation strategy to enhance our financial resource retirement opportunities. Mary identified three timeshare properties that MDI purchased, that gave us flexibility in prime locations where we could travel and vacation very economically.

Mary would research exciting locations for us to travel to each month. It was common that we would visit my sister Shirley and brother-in-law Stan Sykes in Florida, drop in to see my brother Melvin and my sister Joan and their families in St. Louis. We would arrange for a gathering of Mary's brothers and sisters, David, Terry, Mona, and Margaret Ann, and their families while in the St. Louis area. Mary's nieces and nephews were always available to come together to see their aunt Pookie and Uncle Willis.

Mary's adult cousins, Jo Jo (Ardella), Linda, René, Corliss, and her other Byas family members, were certain to engage "Pookie" for catch-up time. Also, we would travel to Los Angeles to visit with our West Coast family; and take a weekend trip during the summer to Las Vegas.

Mary would invite my sister Jean (Drake) to come visit her for her birthday every year. We would celebrate Mary's birthday at Phillips restaurant in Washington DC. They would feast on crab legs, and finished their meal with cake and ice cream. They would go shopping, to wrap up a wonderful birthday celebration. Mary truly enjoyed spending her birthday with Jean.

Additionally, we would host our West Coast family members annually during Christmas week in Palm Springs, California. We reserved one or two timeshare units and provided food for the gathering. My cousin, Don Drake, and his wife, Linda, would also visit us in Palm Springs during that time. Their sons Derrick, Darrell, and Dermar always made time available to visit with us as well. We would visit our great-niece Tamiko Hairston-Hunter, her husband Kelvin & their son KJ in Phoenix, Arizona, annually too.

Our retirement routine was consistent from 2004 until 2011. Month after month, Mary and I enjoyed a gala-like experience, being together, and living our retirement years as senior citizens. Then suddenly, without any cautionary warning, what had been a normal day became very emotional and frightening.

Mary had not been feeling the greatest for several days. However, she rarely would complain regardless of not feeling one hundred percent. On this particular day, the weather outside was a little chilly still, and we were lingering around in the family room.

Mary seemed to be in a state of malaise, and I was concerned to the point that I asked if she wanted to see the doctor. She hunched her shoulders up and down, saying, "I don't know; I just don't feel right! Baby, I feel listless, just no energy."

However, I don't think I can see the doctor today. I said why don't you call the doctor's office anyway. When the new female doctor joined the three male doctors' practice, Mary switched for the female physician to be her primary doctor. In a short time, they established a trustworthy doctor-patient relationship.

When Mary called the doctor's office, she agreed for Mary to come in without an appointment. I drove Mary to the doctor's office, and, seeing the doctor, Mary explained, "I just don't feel that well. I can't say anything hurts me, but I don't have any energy." The doctor gave Mary a regular physical examination, and then she ordered blood tests (Lab work) to be done.

After her examination, I was in the room with Mary and her doctor. In her congenial way, the doctor painstakingly explained to Mary that she could not find anything physically wrong with her that would cause her to feel so fatigued.

The doctor patted Mary's hand. Saying, "the lab work would determine if something internally was going on with you. She explained that possibly there might be toxins in your system, so I am referring you to a Nephrologist, Dr. Kourosh Dibadj, MD, for further examination, and I want you to make an appointment immediately.

Mary, with a forced smile, but concern permeated her face, and she said, "okay, doctor, I will call and make an appointment as soon as I get home. Driving home, it was obvious that Mary was now worried. She said, "I hope nothing is wrong with my kidneys." When we got home, Mary called and made an appointment for the next day with Dr. Dibadj.

Prior to her appointment, Mary's stamina didn't change, and her level of fatigue was persistent. I took Mary to her appointment at Dr. Dibadj's office.

Neither Mary nor I were specifically familiar with the Fairfax, VA area. However, it only took twenty-five minutes to arrive at the doctor's office. We entered the office, and a friendly receptionist asked if we had an appointment.

Mary said, "she was a new patient, and her appointment with Dr. Kourosh Dibadj was at 10 o'clock. The receptionist gave Mary the necessary administrative paperwork to fill out, and she completed the forms and was ready to see the doctor rather quickly. I accompanied Mary to the doctor's consultation room, and when Dr. Dibadj came in, he introduced himself and shook both Mary's and my hand.

He was affable, and physically he appeared to be about five feet nine inches tall, slightly built and weighing about one hundred sixty pounds. He had dark black hair and a light brown skin complexion. He was very professional and compassionate as he informed Mary that she had kidney failure.

Looking at Mary's face, I immediately retreated deep into my memory. I recalled, notably, the two situations she had encountered in past years that struck a nerve with me. One was "The conversation" that Mary and I had and the "vindication" of her unjust job termination. Therefore I knew we would overcome this monumental challenge together, knowing as well that God would provide.

It was the winter of 2011 when Dr. Dibadj gave Mary the only option she had. He informed her of the two types of Dialysis treatments, Hemodialysis and Peritonea Dialysis. He explained that she had to go on Hemo dialysis treatment immediately. What if she chooses peritoneal dialysis later? It will take six to eight weeks to insert a device (port) to allow her to start the peritoneal dialysis treatment.

On February 28, 2011, Mary started her Hemo Dialysis treatment at the Davita Dialysis Clinic located at 2751 Killarney Drive, Woodbridge, VA 22192. Her dialysis appointments were Monday, Wednesday, and Friday at 4:30 pm. Mary needed a wheelchair for her mobility and a taxicab service to transport her.

Mr. Chad Sterling had just started working as a taxicab driver for the Yellow Taxicab Company. I am convinced; people and individuals are brought into your life when they are supposed to be there. When Mary started her dialysis treatments, her mobility was restricted, and she used a wheelchair to get around. Therefore, she had to be transported in a taxicab van.

When Mary first started going to the Davita Dialysis Clinic, the taxicab service was not totally reliable. The cab driver often times was late, and that caused Mary's Dialysis treatment to be delayed in some cases. However, when Chad started working for the Yellow Taxicab Company, he became Mary's primary driver. He would pick her up and return her home from the clinic on time. Chad also became like a member of our family.

Other patients at the clinic thought Chad was Mary's son. They often commented on how he assisted me in getting Mary to and from her Dialysis treatments and the attention and care he provided for Mary. Chad attended special family occasions like Mary's birthday celebration and my granddaughter Adriana's college graduation from Georgetown University.

I presented Mr. Chad Sterling on January 16, 2016, a "Letter of Appreciation" as a formal thank you on behalf of my late wife, Mrs. Mary Ann Byas-Drake, and our family. The thoughtfulness and care he displayed in transporting her were exemplary. He basically was her private driver, transporting her to her scheduled weekly appointments at the Davita

Hemo and Peritonea Dialysis Facility and all her scheduled doctor visits and unscheduled hospital visits.

The dialysis treatment lasted three and a half to four hours. So it would be 9:00 o'clock at night when we got home. Also, with the Hemo dialysis, our social life and activity as we knew it no longer existed. Every aspect of our lives was focused on the Hemodialysis schedule.

Emotionally Mary was in an exceptionally low spirit during her Hemo dialysis treatments. Restriction-wise, the dialysis schedule caused such limitations. We were used to traveling at least ten months out of the twelve-month calendar year.

Mary and I prayed about it, and we resolved to make the best of the current Hemo dialysis situation; and to pursue the option of Mary having peritoneal dialysis treatment as soon as possible.

Mary was immediately impressed with Dr. Dibadj, and so was I. At the Davita clinic, Mary had terrific Registered Nurses (RN) and dialysis technicians that operated the dialysis equipment. As she became familiar with the staff at the clinic, a friendship developed. Her favorite nurses and professional staff workers were: Gloria Nwadiuko, RN; Jodi Holly-Kestel, RN; Daronda Walsh, RN; Luvan Sarmiento, RN; Kathy Trombly, Social Worker and Sandy Brown-Gregory, Dietitian.

Mary and I both immersed ourselves in researching the benefits of peritoneal dialysis treatment. As we became informed, we learned that peritoneal dialysis is a way to remove waste products from your blood when your kidneys can't adequately do the job any longer. This procedure filters the blood in a unique way than the more common blood-filtering procedure called Hemodialysis.

We consulted with Dr. Dibadj, who approved Mary as a suitable candidate for peritoneal dialysis treatment. During the next approval stage in the process, the lead peritoneal dialysis nurse, Jodi Holly-Kestel, RN, made an on-site visit to inspect our home. She had to evaluate our premises to ensure that Mary could receive safe and sufficient peritoneal dialysis treatment at home.

Following the on-site inspection, our home was approved and certified, and Mary conducted her peritoneal dialysis treatments at home. Amazingly, her emotional spirit was immediately and tremendously uplifted, as was mine. Using the peritoneal dialysis process, the most consequential concern was to prevent Mary from getting an infection.

Like switching on a light, we were now able to resume a more normal lifestyle, including traveling. So, in short order, we resumed our traveling schedule. Mary selected the places we would vacation, and I handled the coordination of ensuring that her peritoneal dialysis supplies were ordered in time; to ensure they would arrive concurrently or before we did at the vacation location.

We were now able to function basically as we had before Mary was on dialysis. It was a team effort, Mary was doing her part, and I did mine. We planned our activities from early morning until nighttime as we engaged in the activities we enjoyed. Our travels turned into a means of highlighting how individuals at the Davita Clinic that were on peritoneal dialysis could travel freely in a very normal manner.

Mary became the model peritoneal dialysis "poster patient." In concert with our travels, Jodi Holly-Kestel, RN, created a map of the United States and the Caribbean islands and displayed it on their bulletin board at the clinic. Jodi asked Mary to take pictures of the places we traveled to, and she would post the pictures on the bulletin board map, showing where we had traveled that month. Each month we gave Jodi pictures to display on her bulletin board.

With Mary's participation, Jodi's campaign to encourage her other peritoneal dialysis patients to travel and enjoy life as they had in the past was successful. Several peritoneal dialysis patients also gave Jodi pictures of their travels to display on the bulletin board. Mary was the "poster child" for the Davita clinic peritoneal dialysis, and she served as an inspiration to the other peritoneal dialysis patients.

For many years, before and since our retirement, Mary and I had traveled on vacations with our best friends, Charles and Emma Smith. When Mary started on dialysis, subsequently we decided just the two of us, Mary, and I, would travel together and spend as much time together as possible.

The decision for us to spend our time together is also something that I cannot explain. It was as if I had a spiritual awareness that the time we would share during this time would become invaluable to us personally, day in and day out, over the remaining years of Mary's life.

CHAPTER 41

The Conclusion: Mary's Passing (Transition), December 30, 2015

FOR ELEVEN YEARS (2004 TO 2014), Mary and I enjoyed our retirement lives together. There was not much we wanted to do that we did not actually do. We had the time, we enjoyed one another's company, and we had sustainable resources to undertake the pleasures we enjoyed. However, it's difficult to comprehend how fast our lives would change.

It was July 2014, and we had enjoyed a normal evening, and we went to bed after watching TV as usual. The next morning, Mary was sitting at the kitchen table when I came downstairs. I said good morning, and I kissed her. Then she got up and walked to the laundry room.

A minute later, I heard Mary calling my name loudly, Willis, Willis. It was an excruciating sound as it echoed in the air. Reacting quickly, it only took me 10 steps, and I was in the laundry room, and I was able to catch Mary before she fell to the floor.

In an alarming voice, "what's wrong, baby?" I asked. A faint voice said, "Willis, I don't feel well." Kermit Matthew was in the family room, and I called for him to come to help me get his mother in her chair. He rushed to us, and together we put Mary in the kitchen chair.

Mary said, "I don't know what happened. I just felt lightheaded, like I was going to faint." Immediately I said, "Baby, I'm taking you to the hospital emergency room now." Kermit, help me get your mother in the car. With Mary secured in the car, Kermit said, "I will follow you to the hospital in my car."

We arrived at the hospital's emergency room, and Mary was put in a wheelchair and rushed into the ER triage area, where a doctor examined her. It seemed like hours had passed sitting in the ER visitor's lobby. Finally, Kermit and I were summoned to the ER triage area, where the doctor was examining Mary.

Speaking to us, the doctor chose his words deliberately, stating that "Mary's lab work revealed that she has "Sepsis Shock." Doctor, what does that mean I blurted out? He was direct in revealing his prognosis. Calmly, he said, "your wife has an infection; a toxic bacteria was released into her blood system, and it had spread throughout her body."

The doctor then held Mary's right hand in both of his hands, telling her, "The only alternative to save her life was to amputate your left leg above the knee. I was holding Mary's left hand, and she immediately said, "no, no I don't want my leg amputated." Looking directly into my eyes, she said Willis, I don't want my leg cut off."

I gripped Mary's hand tighter, telling her I love you, I love you, and I want you to be alive. Kermit Matthew also pleaded, emphasizing that we did not want to be without her; we wanted her to live, and the only alternative was to amputate her leg to remove the poison from her body. With trepidation, Mary decided that living was our family's best situation, and she agreed to have her leg amputated.

The surgery had to be performed as soon as possible, and we notified our family of Mary's emergency surgery. Family members, including our daughter Monica and Mary's sister Mona, traveled to Virginia and were at the hospital praying for a successful surgery.

On the day of the surgery, it seemed to take forever, and finally, the doctor appeared in the visitor's waiting room and informed us that the operation was successful and Mary was resting well. The family was able to see Mary briefly; then Monica, Adriana, and Mona were able to return to their homes, knowing that Mary would be fine.

Mary remained at the Sentara Hospital, recuperating in the rehab program for a month following her surgery. For the next phase of her rehab and recovery, she was transferred to a rehab facility in Richmond, Virginia, ninety-five miles from our home, due to her requiring dialysis treatments.

I stayed in Richmond at the local Holiday Inn Hotel for two months, being at Mary's bedside from 7 am to 7 pm every day that she was at the rehab facility. Then Mary was transferred to a rehab center in Northern Virginia. Eventually, she was transferred to a rehab center in Burke, Virginia, which was closer to our home.

During her rehab, Mary was blessed with having a dynamic Physical Therapist, Keley Kauk-Cofield, who motivated her, and Mary progressed sufficiently, and she was able to return to our home, where I was able to take care of her. I had the help of a certified caregiver, Nana Akosua Asante, who is a CNA (Certified Nurses Aid).

Keley continued giving Mary physical therapy twice weekly in our home, and Mary's progress was ongoing. The day before her birthday, "Rishan," Mary's beautician, came to the house and fixed her hair. Mary's "Fro" was tight, and she looked beautiful, just like when her Aunt Biddy use to fix her hair.

On October 15, at 5:00 pm, we celebrated Mary's 74th birthday with family and friends at our home. I was at Mary's side with Willis Jr. (Birdie), Marilyn; Monica and Adriana; Kermit Matthew, Danita, and Déjà. Also, our friends. Charles and Emma Smith; Chad Sterling; Nana Akosua Asante and her children Jared Asante-Wireko, and her daughter Jolyne-Marie (JoJo).

I had baked Mary her favorite yellow cake with chocolate icing; I also bought her a helium-inflated "Happy Birthday balloon" for her birthday. We gathered around the kitchen table and sang happy birthday to Mary. Her granddaughter Déjà helped her grandmother blow out her birthday candles.

Her "Happy Birthday Balloon" was inflated and suspended in air, with a string and a weight to keep the balloon from floating up to the ceiling. In our family tradition, Mary had the first slice of her birthday cake and a scoop of ice cream. That was a happy occasion for Mary and our family, and the smile on Mary's face reflected her beautiful inner spirit.

We recorded on video Mary's 74th birthday celebration. In the video footage, Mary's Happy Birthday Balloon is clearly visible, inflated, and floating on a string suspended in the air. Now it was four weeks after Mary's birthday, and her balloon was still inflated and suspended in the air. In my experience, seeing a balloon inflated this long, four weeks, was an anomaly.

I was at the Dollar General store, and out of curiosity, I asked the store manager if she knew, on average, the length of time that a helium-inflated birthday balloon would stay inflated and suspended in the air.

For a minute, there was a quizzical look on her face. Then she said emphatically, "normally, these balloons probably stay inflated for a week or two weeks at the longest. Driving home, I thought about what the store manager had said: usually, the balloons would only stay inflated for a few weeks.

Historically, when I observe something occurring that is beyond what is normal. I recognize that there is a possible spiritual element involved, or there could be a miraculous situation at hand. However, the reality of Mary's Happy Birthday balloon gives creditability that a spiritual element was involved.

Our daily routine continued as normal with Mary's dialysis schedule and our regular daily activities each day. Mary's physical therapist Keley moved out of state, and we never got another physical therapist of her quality.

In November 2015, Mona and Margaret Ann, Mary's young sisters, paid an emotional visit to their big sister. It was a memorable moment when the three sisters sang a song together that we recorded on video. Also, Mona and Margaret Ann got a big kick out of their big sister, Mary, telling me, "man, be quiet and give me a kiss." The sound of the trio laughing was unique and comical to hear. Happiness was in the air as Mary immensely enjoyed her young sisters' visit.

Additionally, my sister Jean and Mary had a special sister-in-law bond. Their relationship was more as sisters. It seemed that Mary was anticipating Jean's annual visit around this time of year. It was approaching December 29, 2015, and Mary had asked me several times, is Jean here yet? I told Mary I would be picking Jean up from the airport today, and she would be here this evening.

When Jean arrived at our home Tuesday afternoon, she went straight to Mary's bedside. They exchange their usual pleasantries, holding hands and laughing as they always did. The evening passed in a state of gaiety as we retired for the night. The next morning I woke Mary up as usual at 8:30, and Nana, the CNA, came to clean Mary up and get her dressed.

Jean came downstairs and immediately greeted Mary, asking if she had rested well last night. Jean fixed a light breakfast and sat at Mary's bedside, laughing and talking like old times. Time passed quickly, and it was now time for Mary's nap. I would take a nap when Mary did, and Jean also took a nap at this time.

I woke up from my nap on Wednesday afternoon, December 30, at approximately 4:00 pm. I went to Mary's bedside, kissed her as I normally did, and then I realized that Mary did not respond as she usually would. I called out, Jean, Jean, "Mary's gone. I know she has gone home to be with our Heavenly Father, Lord God Almighty!"

From this point, I don't recall the exact sequence of things. I contacted Deacon Larry Hester from our church (Antioch Baptist Church, in Fairfax Station, Virginia), and soon afterward, he and my pastor, Dr. Rev. Marshal L. Ausberry, Sr. came to my home and assisted me spiritually.

Mary's expiring was a tremendous loss for me personally, and our collective families and our friends. I loved her dearly, and we had a blessed and happy married life together. We had been married 55 years, eight months, and 15 days when she transitioned to her spiritual existence to be with her heavenly father, Lord God Almighty.

Willis Jr., Monica, Kermit Matthew, and I made arrangements for Mary's "Home Going (Funeral) Service," which was on January 9, 2016, at Antioch Baptist Church. Rev. Dr. Marshal L. Ausberry, Sr., performed her eulogy. Mary, as she had lived her life every day, she had created her eulogy.

Mary's brother-in-law, Rev. Steve Wooten; a childhood friend, Marie Morris (Hurst); a coworker, Percy Norman; a cousin Linda Turner; a niece Shirley Drake-Hairston; and Paula Drake-Miller; Deacon Larry Hester and Rev. James (Jim) Harden, they all provided scripture and warm comments about Mary.

I thought of Mary so deeply after she had passed and was funeralized. My thoughts of her motivated me to discuss with my son Kermit Matthew to create the "Mary Ann Byas-Drake (Pookie); A Beautiful Life, DVD Video."

I selected particular photos and video footage that I had of Mary during her youthful years, her mature, sophisticated years, as well as her senior citizen years of her life. I incorporated the narrative statements from family and friends that told the story from their perspective of what Mary meant to them. Kermit masterfully incorporated and merged the digitized photo images and videos of his mother into a life-like representation.

The video was completed in late April 2016. I personally provided my sons, Willis Jr. and Kermit Matthew, a copy of the video. Then I flew to

Cleveland, Ohio, to visit my daughter Monica Drake-Zinn at her home in Sagamore Hills, Ohio, and I personally delivered a copy of the DVD Video to Monica in May 2016. The video is registered with the Library of Congress, United States Copyright Office under the registration number: PAu 3-845-842, June 3, 2016.

There is one oddity that existed in the video footage from when we celebrated Mary's seventy-fourth birthday on October 15, 2015, until I completed the video. In the video footage, her Happy Birthday Balloon is visible on a string floating in the air. I was informed that these helium-inflated balloons would normally stay inflated for two weeks at the longest.

In the video, the balloon is now almost deflated. The fact is that Mary's Happy Birthday Balloon stayed inflated from October 15, 2015, until June 7, 2016. It stayed inflated for over **seven months until I had completed making her "Mary Ann Byas-Drake (Pookie) "A Beautiful Life" video.** It was exhilarating, relaxing, cathartic, and therapeutic for me to make "Mary's DVD.

Acknowledgments

To THE MEMORY OF "MARY Ann Byas-Drake" the love of my life and affectionately known to her family as "Pookie" also. The fifty-five wonderful years of marriage we shared and that has sustained me to tell her (our) story. We were spiritually connected and equally yoked. Lord God Almighty blessed us and our family greater than we deserved.

Mary's childhood friends Ceola Lucas, Marie Morris (Hurst), Juanita Rupert (Russell) and Phyllis McNeese-McReynolds. They taught her the value of friendships that guided her throughout her teenager and adult life. Vivian (Vickie) Vaughn, Florence Jean Washington, were HGP nursing classmates that became lifelong friends too.

When we moved to Springfield, Michigan Mary met Mildred Wright, and they bonded immediately. Their friendship evolved into a genuine big sister and little sister relationship, and Mildred's friendship was invaluable to Mary living apart from our family in St. Louis for the first time.

It is worthy to acknowledge Gene and Anne Schumacher and their family. Especially, at that time, their 9 and 7 years old kids, Mary, and Ronnie, that welcomed Willis Jr., and Monica to the neighborhood and were their friends.

I also want to acknowledge the person that edited my manuscript; her profile name is "Accurate Grace." She rendered exceptional editing services that helped make this "Mary's" book interesting and exciting to read!

Definitions and Related Information

References

Climbing the Ladder, Chasing the Dream; The History of Homer G. Phillips Hospital (Author: Candace O'Connor) Chapter nine, page 177, Minnie E. T. Gore. (Note 1).

"In 1951, a new director of nursing was appointed: Miss Minnie E. T. Gore, who had previously served as a staff nurse, head nurse, medical supervisor, and assistant superintendent of nursing at the hospital. A firm believer in advanced education for nurses, she sees herself having a bachelor's degree in nursing education, plus a Master's degree and some work toward a doctorate. She proved to be a powerful force in the hospital's history. While some students found her daunting or even unfriendly, others describe her as strong but fair and often very kind."

Chapter Eleven, pages 237–238, Minnie E. T. Gore. (Note 2).

A handful got special dispensation to marry during training. "Our class was the first that they allowed to get married," said Alverne Meekins Eldridge, class of 1966, "and I was fortunate to get married at the beginning of my senior year." But the administration may have been keen observers of relationships. "Curtis is my ex-husband, and we got married while I was still in school, though I was about to graduate," said nurse Carol Horton. "I had to ask Miss. Gore for permission—and her response was to save enough money for the divorce." Page 237–238.

Miss. Minnie Edythe Todd Gore—most alumnae remember her with great respect; page 252.

Miss. Minnie Edythe Todd Gore (1909–1983)—page 253.

Miss. Gore was appointed in 1951 as the director of nursing at HGP (Ch. 12; pg. 83). (The book title: *Climbing the Ladder, Chasing the Dream,* Ch. 11; pg. 237; the author is Candace O'Connor).

Note: Mary Byas-Drake was allowed by Miss. Gore, in 1960, to be married and returned to HGP nursing school. This predates the decision that "A handful (students) got special dispensation to marry during training." Our class was the first that they allowed to get married," said a student in the class of 1966." (Ch. 12; pg. 85). (The book title: *Climbing the Ladder, Chasing the Dream,* Ch. 11; pg. 237; the author is Candace O'Connor).

Homer G. Phillips Hospital:
https://en.wikipedia.org/wiki/Homer_G._Phillips_Hospital

Homer G. Phillips Nurses Dormitory (2516 Goode Avenue)
Note 1: https://www.bing.com/images

Validated Information

1. I had firsthand knowledge from past experiences of my mother's visions being manifested and fulfilled. My mother's blessing of receiving visions from the "Holy Spirit is documented in my first book titled "I Missed The Bus, But I Arrived On Time!"

2. Mary was inducted into the RHO chapter, University of Michigan, Ann Arbor, Michigan, April 16, 1985, as a member of the National Honor Society of Nursing "Sigma Theta Tau"

3. The church I am a member is: Antioch Baptist Church, 6531 Little Ox Road, Fairfax Station, VA, ZIP Code 22039.